POCKET
FIRST AID

British Red Cross Society
in association with
Dorling Kindersley Publishers Limited

Text and illustrations advisors
The British Red Cross Society

Brigadier D.D. O'Brien *Chief Medical Officer*

Miss M.E. Baker *Director of Training*

Mr J. Williams *Training Department*

Editor
Jemima Dunne

Art Editor
Julia Harris

Senior Art Editor
Anne-Marie Bulat

Managing Editor
Daphne Razazan

First published in Great Britain in 1985 by
Dorling Kindersley Publishers Limited,
9 Henrietta Street, Covent Garden, London WC2E 8PS.
Reprinted 1988, 1990

British Library Cataloguing in Publication Data
Pocket first aid
   1. First aid in illness and injury
   I. Red Cross, *British Red Cross Society*
   616.02'52   RC87

ISBN 0-86318-010-8

CONTENTS

PRINCIPLES OF FIRST AID

What is first aid?

First aid is the first assistance or treatment given to an injured person (casualty) before the arrival of an ambulance or qualified expert.

What are the objectives of first aid?

The three objectives of first aid are to:
- Preserve life.
- Prevent the injury or condition worsening.
- Promote recovery.

How is this done?

Your task as a First Aider is to:
- Find out what happened without endangering your own life.
- Reassure and protect the person from any further danger.
- Arrange for travel home or to the nearest hospital as necessary.

What equipment is needed?

You do not need any special equipment. First-aid kits do contain many useful items such as dressings and bandages but a good first aider should not rely on them. You should use whatever is readily available, improvising if necessary.

DEALING WITH AN EMERGENCY

When dealing with any emergency your approach is one of the most important factors. You must remain calm and confident while you assess the situation and carry out any necessary treatment. This will reassure everyone and convince them of your ability to cope.

Hazards

It is very important that when attempting to rescue a casualty you do not become a casualty yourself. Some incidents are particularly dangerous, for instance, if the casualty is still in contact with electricity, near a fire or in a room filled with poisonous fumes. In *any* of these situations you must take certain safety precautions before you do anything (see pp. 10–11).

Golden rules to remember

We have used a home accident to help demonstrate the necessary procedures (see overleaf) but the same rules apply to any incident:

● Do not approach the casualty if doing so will put your life in danger;
● Always attend to the most seriously injured person first;
● Never move a casualty unless absolutely necessary (i.e., if his or her life is in immediate danger).

What to do

If there is an accident in or around your home, follow the procedures described on the following pages and apply any first aid treatments as necessary by referring to the *A–Z of First Aid* on pages 33 to 82. Remember, use your common sense, know your limitations and do not attempt too much.

HOW TO HANDLE AN ACCIDENT

IMPORTANT

● Never touch a casualty who is still in contact with electricity (see p. 10).
● Always remove the danger from the casualty and only move the casualty from the danger if this is not possible.
● Never leave an unconscious person alone.

WHAT TO DO

1 Look around you. Try to find out what happened – if the casualty is conscious she should be able to tell you.

2 Make sure that there is no further danger. There may be something about to fall on the person, a drill may still be switched on or there may be a fire nearby.

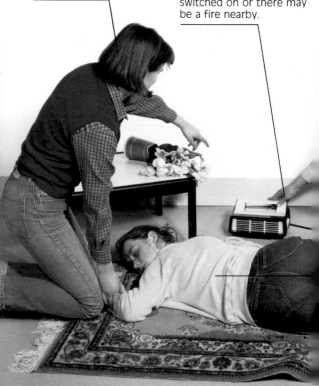

Other points to look for

Careful observation of the history of the incident and any symptoms and signs of injury will help you to know what treatment the casualty will need.

● **History** How did it happen? Ask the casualty or casualties and anyone else who saw the incident.

● **Symptoms** Listen very carefully to everything the casualty tells you. Is she in pain, where is the pain? Is she unable to move, why can't she move?

● **Signs** Gently examine the casualty from head to foot. What can you see and feel – is she breathing, is she blue, is she conscious, is there any bleeding, is there any deformity in the limbs (compare one side of the body with the other), is the pulse weak, is she very pale? In addition, look out for any medical warning signs such as a Medic-alert bracelet or S.O.S. Talisman.

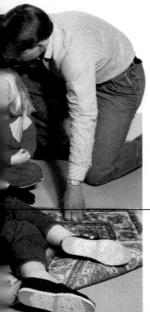

3 If there is more than one casualty, quickly decide which is the most seriously injured and treat her according to the priorities listed overleaf.

4 Send for an ambulance or doctor as required, giving accurate details about the accident (see *Calling for help*, p. 9).

! PRIORITIES

The priorities for treatment of any casualty are listed below. However, in all incidents where there are several casualties, the most severely injured person should always be treated first. But remember, the noisy casualty may not be the most severely injured.

WHAT TO DO

1 A.B.C. must be established immediately if the casualty is unconscious in order to prevent permanent injury – brain damage can occur after only three minutes without oxygen.

A is for AIRWAY. The passage between the mouth, nose, throat and windpipe (*the airway*) must be kept open and clear (see pp. 20–1).

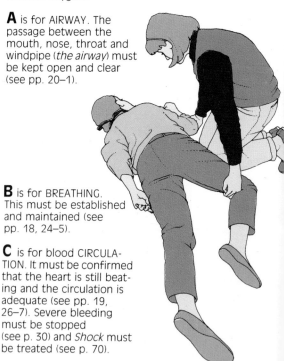

B is for BREATHING. This must be established and maintained (see pp. 18, 24–5).

C is for blood CIRCULA-TION. It must be confirmed that the heart is still beating and the circulation is adequate (see pp. 19, 26–7). Severe bleeding must be stopped (see p. 30) and *Shock* must be treated (see p. 70).

2 Broken bones must be immobilised if the casualty is to be moved (see pp. 37–43). Do not move a casualty with a suspected back or neck injury (see p. 35).

3 Reassure the casualty and treat any other injuries as required according to *A–Z of First Aid* pages 33–82.

CALLING FOR HELP

Throughout this book we recommend that you refer a casualty to medical aid if you are in any doubt about his or her condition. Medical aid means treatment by a doctor.

Ambulances are normally needed to take a casualty to hospital from *all* serious outdoor accidents and *any* incident involving: difficulty in breathing, heart failure, severe bleeding, unconsciousness, serious burns, suspected broken bones (although a casualty with a broken arm can normally be taken by car), shock or poisoning.

Calling the emergency services

If possible always stay with the casualty and ask someone else to telephone for the ambulance. However, if you will be able to see the casualty from the telephone, you can make the call yourself following steps 1 to 5 below. If another person makes the call, ask them to come back and tell you that the call has been made.

WHAT TO DO

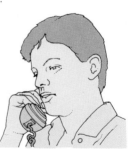

1 Dial 999 and ask for the appropriate emergency service (normally ambulance because each switchboard has access to all the others and the control officer can notify the other services).

2 Give the operator your telephone number just in case you are cut off.

3 Give details of: the exact location of the accident (describe any landmarks the ambulance driver may need to find the house or area); what happened and the suspected cause; the number, sex and approximate age of the casualties involved; and the extent of the injuries.

4 Listen very carefully to the control officer. He or she may tell you what to do while you are waiting for the ambulance to arrive.

5 Do not replace the telephone receiver before the ambulance control officer does so.

9

ELECTRICITY

If the casualty is still in contact with electricity, STOP THE CURRENT at once by switching it off at the mains or pulling out the plug. If this is not possible, knock the casualty's limb clear of the electrical contact as shown below. *Do not attempt to give first aid or to touch the casualty until the contact has been broken.*

IMPORTANT

Do not touch the casualty with anything wet because water conducts electricity.

Breaking the contact

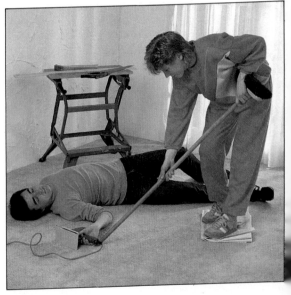

1 Stand on a dry surface, for example, on a rubber mat, newspaper or a piece of wood.

2 Knock the casualty's limb away from the object using the end of a wooden broom handle or something made of a similar non-conductive material (i.e., not metal).

FIRES

If you are confronted by a fire at home, or in the street, act quickly and precisely. Do not enter a burning building alone. Not only is there a danger of your being overcome by smoke, but also, as fire spreads very quickly, you may be burnt yourself. Moreover, a great deal of modern furniture is made of materials that give off toxic fumes when burning: these fumes can kill in a matter of seconds. If you are in a building and discover a fire, act as described here.

WHAT TO DO

1 Close the door of the room with the fire; *do not enter the room.*

2 Alert everyone in the house to the danger and get them out of the building by the safest route; *if you live in a block of flats, do not use the lift.*

3 Call the fire brigade (see p. 9) giving as much detail as possible and tell the neighbours of the danger.

4 If you are cut off by fire, go into a room with a window and SHUT the door. Put a blanket or something similar along the bottom of the door to stop the smoke entering the room, open the window and call for help.

Chip-pan fires

When using a chip pan or deep fryer, make sure that it is never more than half full and never leave the pan without turning it off. If a chip pan catches fire, NEVER pour water on it – it will explode and the fire will spread.

What you should do
Turn off the heat and smother the flames with the saucepan lid or a damp cloth and leave it covered for at least half an hour.

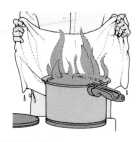

MOVING A CASUALTY

The casualty's comfort and well-being should always be your first consideration and this is particularly so if you have to move someone. Remember the golden rules:

● The danger should be removed from the casualty and only if this is not possible should you move the casualty from the danger.

● Never try to move a person by yourself if there are other people available to help.

Do not make the injury worse

Always wait for skilled help to arrive; careless handling of the casualty can make an injury much worse. For example, a broken bone could pierce a blood vessel and cause serious internal bleeding. Therefore, if for any reason the casualty has to be moved, you must immobilise the joints above and below any suspected broken bone, by hand or with padding and bandages or slings (see pp. 37–43), and/or apply direct pressure to control bleeding (see p. 30) before you do so.

Which method to use

There are various ways to move a person described on the following pages; the method you use will depend on the injury, the number of people available to help, the casualty's build, and the route to be travelled. A stretcher will always be needed to move a seriously injured or ill person and will be brought by the ambulance.

Principles of lifting

If you observe the following rules carefully, you will find yourself able to lift heavy objects without undue strain. Try to practise these techniques so that you are prepared in an emergency. However, do not practise lifting anything or anyone heavier than yourself.

● Stand with your feet slightly apart.

● Keep your back straight; always bend the knees

● Keep the weight close to your body.

● Use your thighs, hips and shoulders – the most powerful muscles of your body – to take as much of the weight as possible.

MOVING A CASUALTY TO SAFETY

If danger such as the possibility of fire makes it
necessary to move a casualty to safety very
quickly, use the following method.

WHAT TO DO

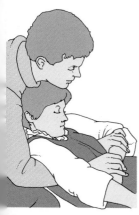 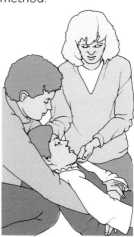

1 Crouch behind the
casualty. Fold one of
her arms across her chest
(make sure it is uninjured).
Slide your arms beneath
her armpits and grasp the
casualty's arm.

2 If possible, ask someone to help steady her
head and neck to keep
them in line with her body.
Then both of you should
move slowly backwards
dragging the casualty.

CARRYING LIGHT CASUALTIES

There are two ways of carrying injured children
and light adults. You can cradle them in your arms
or carry them pick-a-back fashion.

Cradle method
Squat down beside the
casualty and pass one arm
under her thighs and the
other around her back and
lift. *Do not use this
method if the casualty has
a back injury or a broken
leg.*

Pick-a-back
Squat with your back to
the casualty and tell her
to put her arms around
your neck and clasp her
hands together at the
front. Put your arms
around her legs and stand
up. *This method cannot be
used if limbs are broken.*

HELPING THE CASUALTY TO WALK

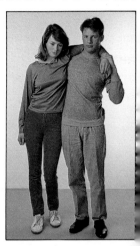

This method is used to help support a casualty who is able to walk. It should *never be used if an arm is injured*. If the casualty needs more help ask another person to support the other side.

What to do
Stand at the casualty's injured side and put the arm nearest you around your neck and hold on to her hand. Put your other arm around her waist and grab hold of her clothing at her hip and walk slowly.

TWO-HANDED SEAT

This method requires two people and is used if a person cannot walk and has a chest or arm injury.

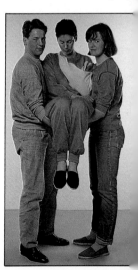

WHAT TO DO

1 Squat facing each other on either side of the casualty and each pass an arm around the casualty's back and grasp her clothing on the side farthest from you.

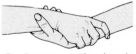

2 Pass your other hands under the thighs and grasp each other's wrists.

3 Gently raise the casualty and set off leading with your outside foot take normal paces.

!

CHAIR SUPPORT

If you have to move a casualty along a narrow passage or up or down stairs, you can seat him or her in a chair and carry the chair with the help of another person. Before you start, make sure the chair can take the casualty's weight and clear any obstructions or loose mats out of the way.

WHAT TO DO

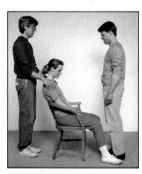

1 Sit the casualty on the chair. Stand behind the chair and ask your helper to stand in front facing the casualty.

2 Make sure the casualty is sitting well back in the chair. For additional safety, secure her with **broad-fold bandages** (see p. 86).

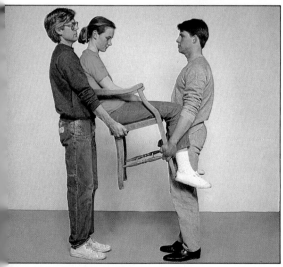

3 Support the back of the chair and the casualty while your helper holds the front legs. Working together, tip the chair back slightly and lift it. With the casualty facing forward, move along the passage.

15

FIRST-AID KITS

Although you can improvise in an emergency it is always better to have a fully equipped first-aid kit at home. The list of items to keep in a first-aid kit suggested below, is based on equipment used in the book. You will find detailed descriptions of the dressings and bandages, with instructions on how to use them on pages 83–94.

Keep all the equipment in a clean, dry, airtight box. Label the box clearly and keep it in a dry place – preferably not the bathroom because it could be affected by steam. Keep the first-aid kit out of reach of children.

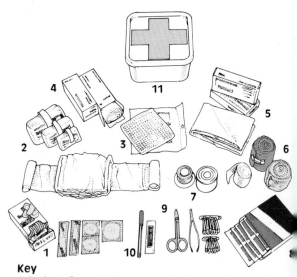

Key

1 Packet of assorted waterproof adhesive dressings (see p. 85).
2 Sterile unmedicated dressings – large, medium and small (see p. 84).
3 Packet of gauze squares.
4 Roll of cotton wool.
5 Triangular bandages – for slings and securing dressings (see p. 88).
6 Roller bandages – open-weave for securing dressings and crepe for supporting joint and muscle injuries (see p. 86).
7 Roll of porous surgical tape – for securing large dressings.
8 Pack of antiseptic wipes
9 Tweezers, scissors and safety pins.
10 Thermometer or temperature indicator strip.
11 Plastic container.

LIFE-SAVING TECHNIQUES

It has been explained in the first section *Dealing with an emergency* that your priority in any accident is to maintain a casualty's vital needs – Airway, Breathing and Circulation. This is important because every part of the body uses oxygen for life and energy; the brain needs more than any other part. Air contains oxygen, so each time we breathe, we take oxygen into our bodies through our mouth and nose. The air passes down the windpipe and into the lungs, from where the oxygen is picked up by the blood and carried to the body tissues where it is needed (see p. 19).

What can go wrong

If there is not enough oxygen available to the tissues, *asphyxia* will occur. This can happen because: there is not enough oxygen in the air (for example, in a smoke-filled garage); the air passages are blocked; or there is interference with, or paralysis of, the muscle action of the chest (for example, if a person is buried under a fall of sand or after an electric shock).

What you can do

The correct use of the techniques described on the following pages will enable you to save lives by keeping the casualty's airway open (*Opening the airway* and *Clearing the airway*) and maintaining the casualty's breathing (*Mouth-to-mouth ventilation*) and circulation (*External chest compression*) until skilled help arrives. See page 30 for a summary of when to use these life-saving techniques. The most important thing to remember before you start is that you must make sure that, by approaching a casualty or accident, you are not putting your own life in danger.

CHECKING BREATHING

Breathing is the process by which air containing oxygen is taken into the lungs and carbon dioxide, a waste product, is expelled from the body.

How we breathe
To breathe, we use the muscles between our ribs and the diaphragm (a dome-shaped muscle that separates the chest from the upper part of the abdomen) to expand our chests and draw air into the lungs. To breathe out, the muscles relax, causing the chest to fall back into the resting position, driving the used air back out of the body through the mouth and nose. Normally, we breathe in and out about 16 times per minute. To find out whether or not an unconscious person is breathing, look along the chest and listen and feel for breathing as shown below.

WHAT TO DO

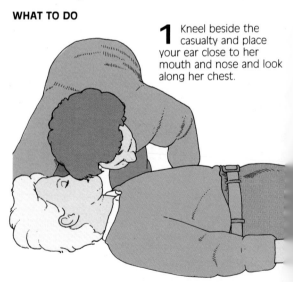

1 Kneel beside the casualty and place your ear close to her mouth and nose and look along her chest.

2 If she is breathing, you will see the chest moving and feel and hear the breaths against the side of your face.

3 If she is not breathing you must **open and clear the airway** (see pp. 20–1), and if necessary begin **mouth-to-mouth** (see p. 24).

CHECKING CIRCULATION

Blood consists of cells suspended in a fluid called plasma. It is pumped by the heart through arteries to every part of the body and returns to the heart in the veins. It carries oxygen (from the lungs), nourishment (from the digested food) and warmth to the body tissues and carries waste products away.

What is a pulse?

When the heart beats a throb passes along every artery. This is known as the pulse and it can be felt anywhere an artery lies close to the surface, for example at the neck (*carotid pulse*) or at the wrist (*radial pulse*). The heart beats 60–80 times per minute. A normal pulse is regular and strong. If there is no pulse, the heart has stopped beating (*cardiac arrest*); if it is fast and weak, the casualty may be in *Shock* (see p. 70).

Carotid pulse

1 Find the casualty's voice box and slide the pads of three fingers into the hollow between it and the large neck muscle.

2 Feel for the pulse for about five seconds. Use this method to find out whether or not a person's heart is beating.

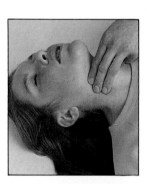

Radial pulse

1 Place the pads of three fingers in the hollow above the creases on the front of a person's wrist in line with the thumb pad.

2 Count the number of beats you can feel in a minute. Use this method to establish the pulse rate of a conscious casualty.

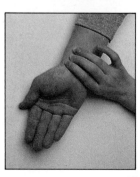

OPENING THE AIRWAY

As we have explained in the introduction to this section, breathing is essential to life. However, breathing is possible only if the space between the nose and mouth and the windpipe (the airway) is open and clear.

What causes a blocked airway?
The danger of airway obstruction is acute if a person is unconscious, and particularly so if he or she is lying face upwards. This is because when a person loses consciousness, the muscles of the jaw relax and the tongue falls back and blocks the throat. In addition, vomit, for example, may collect at the back of the throat, which can also block the casualty's airway.

An unconscious casualty

Tongue fallen back

Vomit at back of throat

Blocked airway

WHAT TO DO

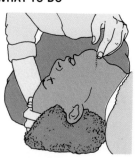

1 Place one hand on the casualty's forehead.

2 With the other hand, push the casualty's lower jaw forward so that the chin juts out. This moves the tongue forward and opens the airway.

3 Look, listen and feel to see if the casualty is breathing (see p.18). If he is, place him in the **recovery position** (see p.22).

CLEARING THE AIRWAY

If the casualty is still not breathing after the airway has been opened, it may be because the airway is blocked, for example, by broken teeth, mud or vomit. You should then clear the casualty's airway as shown below.

If the casualty is conscious, the airway can sometimes be cleared by backslaps, see treatment for *Choking* on page 48.

WHAT TO DO

1 Turn the casualty's head to one side and with one quick sweep round the casualty's mouth with your index finger, carefully lift out any foreign matter.

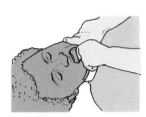

2 Make sure that by doing this you do not push the object further down the casualty's throat.

If the head cannot be turned

If you suspect a fractured neck (see p. 35), or if the casualty is trapped in an upright position, and is not breathing or is making gurgling sounds, *do not turn the head to one side or extend the neck.* Open and clear the airway as described below.

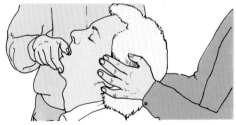

1 Ask a bystander to support the casualty's head. Grasp the lower jaw with one hand and pull it forward; the tongue will automatically come forward with the jaw.

2 Quickly sweep round the casualty's mouth and throat as above and hook out any foreign matter you find in the mouth.

RECOVERY POSITION

All unconscious casualties who are breathing should be placed in the *recovery position*. It keeps them stable in a position which ensures that the airway stays open and that any vomit or secretions can drain freely from the mouth.

Before you place a casualty in the recovery position you must make sure that he or she is breathing normally and that the heart is beating. Then examine him or her for any signs of *back or neck injury* (see p. 32), or *broken bones* (see p. 34). Broken bones must be immobilised before you turn the casualty. Do not turn the casualty if you suspect a back injury; refer to pages 32–3.

IMPORTANT

Never leave an unconscious casualty alone even when he or she has been placed in the recovery position.

WHAT TO DO

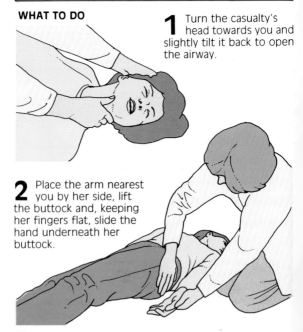

1 Turn the casualty's head towards you and slightly tilt it back to open the airway.

2 Place the arm nearest you by her side, lift the buttock and, keeping her fingers flat, slide the hand underneath her buttock.

3 Gently raise the leg farthest from you and cross it over the near one at the ankle. Then bring the other arm up and lay it across her chest, so that the hand is touching the opposite shoulder.

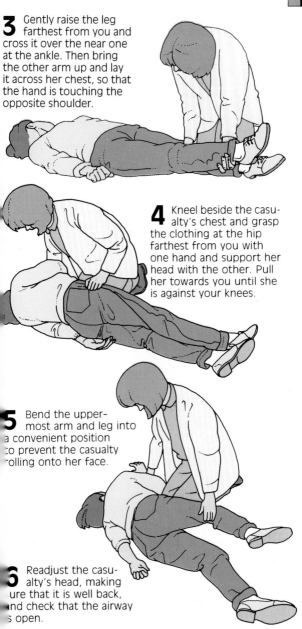

4 Kneel beside the casualty's chest and grasp the clothing at the hip farthest from you with one hand and support her head with the other. Pull her towards you until she is against your knees.

5 Bend the uppermost arm and leg into a convenient position to prevent the casualty rolling onto her face.

6 Readjust the casualty's head, making sure that it is well back, and check that the airway is open.

23

MOUTH-TO-MOUTH VENTILATION

If the casualty is still not breathing after the airway has been opened and cleared, you must load his or her blood with oxygen by breathing air from your lungs into the casualty's mouth (or nose). This is possible because you use only about a quarter of the oxygen you breathe in – the rest is breathed out. This life-saving technique is commonly known as *mouth-to-mouth*.

WHAT TO DO

1 Open and clear the airway. Keep the head back, the jaw forward and the mouth open.

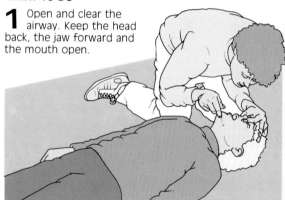

2 Pinch the casualty's nostrils shut with the fingers and thumb of one hand and support the jaw with the other – keep your fingers clear of the mouth and off the throat.

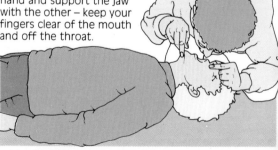

3 Take a deep breath, open your mouth wide and seal your lips around the casualty's mouth. Blow gently but firmly into his mouth.

4 Lift your mouth away from the casualty's and turn your head towards his chest. If you have been successful, you will see that his chest has risen and is falling as the air comes out.

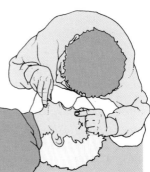

5 Give one more breath to load his blood with oxygen; his skin colour should improve.

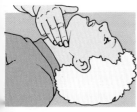

6 Pause and check the casualty's **carotid pulse** (see p. 19).

7 If the heart is beating, continue giving breaths of mouth-to-mouth at a rate of one every three to four seconds; check the pulse again every three minutes.

8 If there is no pulse, begin **external chest compression** (see p. 26).

9 When breathing returns, place the casualty in the **recovery position** (see p. 22).

Mouth-to-nose ventilation

You can blow air into the casualty's nose instead of the mouth.

Forming the seal
Close the casualty's mouth with your thumb and seal your lips around her nose. Continue as in steps 3 to 9 above.

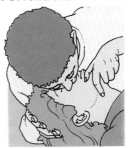

25

EXTERNAL CHEST COMPRESSION

If the casualty is still not breathing after the airway has been opened and cleared and mouth-to-mouth has been started, you must check the blood circulation. Blood is pumped around the body by the heart. If the heart stops circulating the blood, oxygen will not reach the body cells; permanent brain damage can result after only three minutes without oxygen.

What you should do

Check the **carotid pulse** (see p. 19). If there is no pulse (beating), it means that the heart has stopped (cardiac arrest) and you must begin to pump it artificially using *external chest compression*. This involves applying pressure to the lower half of the breastbone, which in turn causes blood to be pushed out of the heart; when you release the pressure, the heart refills.

IMPORTANT

This technique must be taught by a trained instructor and should be practised only on a resuscitation dummy.

WHAT TO DO

1 Lay the casualty on his back on a firm surface. Kneel alongside him facing his chest and in line with his heart. Find the junction of his rib margins at the bottom of his breastbone. Place the heel of one hand along the line of the breastbone, two finger breadths above point, keeping your fingers off the ribs.

2 Place the heel of your hand on the centre of the lower half of the breastbone, cover it with the other hand and lock your fingers together; keep your hands off the casualty's ribs.

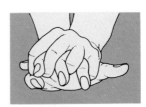

3 Kneel upright so that your shoulders are over the casualty's breast-bone and your arms are straight. Press down about 4.5cm (2in), then release the pressure but do not remove your hands.

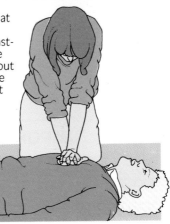

4 Complete 15 compressions at a rate of 80 compressions per minute – count "one-and-two-and-" while you work.

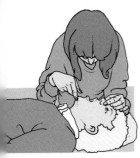

5 When you reach 15, move to the casualty's mouth and give him two breaths of **mouth-to-mouth** (see p. 24).

6 Continue giving 15 compressions follow-ed by 2 breaths of mouth-to-mouth for one minute.

7 Stop and check the **carotid pulse** (see p. 19); check the pulse again every three minutes.

8 When you feel a pulse again, STOP COMPRES-SIONS IMMEDIATELY. Continue with **mouth-to-mouth** alone until breath-ing returns, then place the casualty in the **recovery position** (see p. 22).

TREATING BABIES AND SMALL CHILDREN

The procedures and sequence of steps for opening the airway, mouth-to-mouth and external chest compression are, in principle, the same as for adults. However, the hand positions and breathing and compression rates of some of the techniques must be adapted when treating small children. If a child is conscious and has swallowed a foreign body, he or she may be *Choking*; treat as described on page 48.

You must not use mouth-to-mouth or external chest compression on children unless you have been taught by a trained instructor because incorrect use of either might kill a child.

IMPORTANT

It is dangerous to tilt a baby's head back too far when opening the airway.

Opening the airway

For children aged 2–8 use the technique described on page 20. For babies and small children under 2, treat as described below because their tongues are large, their necks short and their windpipes soft and easily compressed by tilting the head back too far.

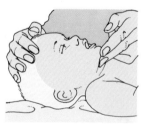

1 Place one hand on the baby's forehead and two fingers of the other hand on the *bony* part of the chin.

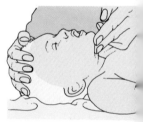

2 Gently press on the forehead and tilt the head back very slightly. Support the chin with the two fingers; *make sure you keep your fingers off the neck*.

Mouth-to-mouth ventilation

For children under 2
Open the airway as des-
cribed opposite. Seal your
lips around the child's
mouth and nose and puff
gently at a rate of about
20 breaths per minute.

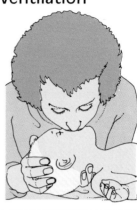

For children aged 2–8
Open the airway, seal your
lips around the child's
mouth (or mouth and
nose according to the size
of the child), and blow
gently at the normal
breathing rate.

IMPORTANT

● Do not over-inflate the lungs; stop blowing
when you see the chest rise.
● Do not press too hard on a child's chest
wall; it is very soft.

External chest compression

For children under 2
Make sure that the child is
on a firm surface. Slide
your hand under the
child's back and support
the head and neck. Place
two fingers over the
centre of the breastbone.
Press down 1.5–2.5cm (½–
1in) and work at a rate of
about 100 compressions
per minute.

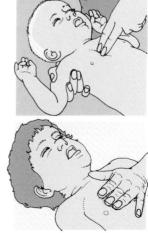

For children aged 2–8
Place the heel of *one hand*
over the centre of the
breastbone. Press down
1.5–3.5cm (1–1½in) and
work at a slightly slower
rate of 80–100 compres-
sions per minute.

29

CONTROLLING SEVERE BLEEDING

Bleeding occurs when any of the vessels that carry blood around the body – arteries, veins or capillaries – are cut or torn. It can be external and visible or internal and invisible (see p. 70). Blood from the arteries is bright red and spurts from a wound; blood from veins is darker red and gushes. Blood from the capillaries is medium-red and oozes from a wound.

Bleeding is an emergency

Serious bleeding is always an emergency because if too much blood is lost from the circulatory system there will not be enough circulating to supply all the body cells with oxygen. *Shock* (see p. 70) and eventually death can result.

WHAT TO DO

1 Raise the affected area. Apply *Direct pressure* to control bleeding by pressing with your fingers or palm of your hand over a clean dressing or pad. If no dressing is immediately available, use your hands. You may need to maintain pressure for up to 15 minutes.

2 If the wound is large, apply pressure gently but firmly above and below the wound and maintain pressure as in step 1 above.

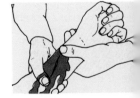

3 Raise and support the injured part so that it is above the level of the casualty's heart (chest). This slows down the blood flow to the injured part; it is called *Elevation*.

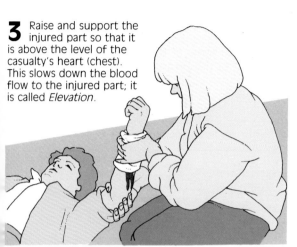

4 Help the casualty to lie down; this will slow the flow of blood down even more.

5 Place a **sterile dressing** (see p. 85) over the wound; it must be large enough to extend well beyond the edges of the wound. Secure it with the attached bandage; tie the knot over the pad.

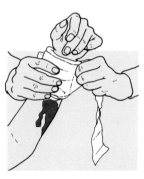

6 If you have no dressing available, use a piece of clean, thick, non-fluffy material instead (see p. 94).

7 If the blood begins to show through the dressing, do not remove the first dressing but put another dressing on top of the first and secure it.

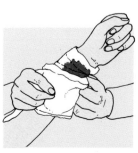

8 Watch for any signs of *Shock* and treat accordingly (see pp. 70–1).

SUMMARY

This chart sets out clearly when to use all the techniques described in this chapter. Do not forget that some of the techniques need to be adapted for use on babies and small children.

IMPORTANT

Do not approach a casualty if doing so puts your life in any danger.

COLLAPSE:
Shake the casualty gently by the shoulders and question him (see p. 76).

IF CONSCIOUS:
Make the casualty comfortable and watch Airway, Breathing and Circulation (pp. 20–1).

IF UNCONSCIOUS:
Check breathing (p. 18). Open the airway (p. 20). Clear the airway (p. 21).

BREATHING:
Turn into recovery position (p. 22). Watch Airway, Breathing and Circulation.

NOT BREATHING
Begin mouth-to-mouth (p. 24) – give 2 breaths. Check carotid pulse (p. 19).

PULSE PRESENT:
Continue mouth-to-mouth until breathing returns – check carotid pulse again every three minutes.

PULSE ABSENT:
Give external chest compression (p. 26) with mouth-to-mouth. Check breathing and pulse after one minute and again every three minutes.

A-Z OF FIRST AID

This section of the book covers first aid for the injuries and conditions you are most likely to come across in and around the home, listed in alphabetical order for easy reference. It includes minor injuries such as *Splinters* and *Small cuts and grazes* as well as more serious injuries such as *Broken bones*, *Burns* and *Head injuries*. In each case we describe the injury or condition with the symptoms and signs and tell you what you can do while you are waiting for medical help to arrive.

Remember the priorities

It cannot be stressed enough that the priority in any accident is to maintain the casualty's vital needs – *Airway*, *Breathing* and *Circulation* (see p. 8). **Open the casualty's airway** (see p. 20), **check breathing** (see p. 18) and make sure the **heart is beating** (see p. 19). Only then should you treat any other injuries you find. This is because the body needs oxygen to survive – vital brain cells will die after only *three* minutes without oxygen.

Multiple injuries

Often the casualty may have two or more injuries. In this situation treatment of one injury may prevent correct treatment of another. Decide which is the most serious injury and treat it as described, then treat other injuries as correctly as possible under the circumstances.

ANIMAL BITES

Animals have sharp, pointed teeth and, because of this, they often leave puncture wounds which inject germs deep into the body tissues, causing infection. Therefore any bite that breaks the skin needs prompt attention to prevent infection developing. In addition, there is a possibility of tetanus infection and in some countries, rabies.

Any incident involving a dog bite should be reported to the police as soon as possible.

Tetanus infection

This is a dangerous infection caused by tetanus germs spreading from a wound into the nervous system and causing severe muscular spasms. The risk of tetanus infection is high if a wound is dirty, deep or contaminated with soil from places where animals graze, or if it contains a foreign body. Everyone can be inoculated and should keep inoculations up to date.

Rabies infection

Rabies is a potentially fatal condition spread by the saliva of infected animals. Although not commonly found in the British Isles, it is endemic in many other countries. If a person is bitten by an animal that could have been smuggled into the country, the police MUST be informed and the casualty will need to have a course of injections.

WHAT TO DO

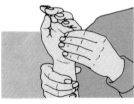

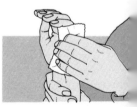

1 Control severe bleeding with **direct pressure** and **elevation** (see p. 30).

2 Clean the wound thoroughly with soap and water (see p. 79).

3 Protect the wound with a **dressing** large enough to cover the area (see pp. 84–5).

4 Seek medical aid; anti tetanus or, in some cases, rabies inoculation may be required.

BACK INJURY

The spine is a column of bones that extends from the skull all the way down the back. It is supported by ligaments and it surrounds and protects the spinal cord – a rope-like structure of nerves – which controls many of the functions of the body. Damage to the spinal cord can result in loss of power, movement and of feeling in parts of the body below the injured area.

Possible injuries

A sudden bending or awkward twisting of the back or neck may strain the muscles of the back; it may result in a sprain of the ligaments supporting the spine; or it may injure the discs between the bones that make up the spine. A direct blow may damage the bones. Suspect a broken spine if, for example, a person has fallen awkwardly or from a height.

WHAT TO DO

1 Tell the casualty not to move. Make her as comfortable as possible in the position in which you find her.

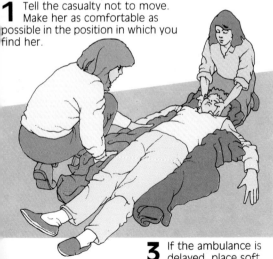

2 Ask someone to steady the casualty's head by hand while you place rolled coats and/or pillows along either side of her body; await the arrival of the ambulance.

3 If the ambulance is delayed, place soft padding between the casualty's legs and tie a **narrow-fold bandage** (see p. 88) around her feet and ankles and a **broad-fold bandage** (see p. 88) around both knees.

B

BLISTERS FROM RUBBING

Blisters develop when skin is damaged by friction or heat; tissue fluid leaks from the damaged area and collects just under the skin. Blisters caused by rubbing, for example, blisters on the heel from a boot or on the hand from digging with a spade, may cause so much discomfort that they need to be treated as described below before you can continue your activity.

IMPORTANT

Never break a blister caused by any form of heat because of the risk of infection (see Burns p. 44).

WHAT TO DO

1 Wipe the blister with cotton wool soaked in methylated spirit, or wash the area with some soap and water.

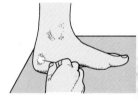

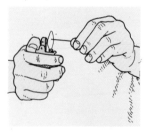

2 Sterilise a needle by passing it through the flame of a match or lighter and allow it to cool. *Do not wipe the soot away or touch the end of the needle for any reason.*

3 Keeping the needle at level of the skin, pass it into the blister in two places; ideally you should make a hole on each side.

4 Place a clean piece of cotton wool on the blister to absorb the fluid.

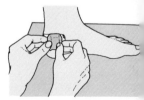

5 Cover the blister with an **adhesive dressing** (see p. 84).

BROKEN BONES

The body is supported by its own scaffolding of bones called the *skeleton*. The bones protect and surround all the vital organs of the body and act as levers for muscles to pull against. Normally bones are strong, but they can break or crack if struck, twisted or bent. Because bones have important blood vessels and organs near them, great care needs to be taken when they break to prevent the organs or blood vessels being damaged by the broken bone ends.

Follow the principles of treatment described below. Special techniques for securing the different bones with padding, slings and/or bandages are described on the following pages.

General symptoms and signs

All the following symptoms and signs may not be present in every case.
● Extreme pain at site of injury – increased by any attempt to move.
● Casualty may have felt or heard a bone snap and may have felt the bone ends grating.
● Swelling and later bruising may develop.
● The affected limb or part of the body may look deformed compared to the other limb or opposite side of the body.
● Symptoms and signs of *Shock* (p. 70).

WHAT TO DO

1 Steady and support the injured part by placing one hand above and one below the injured area.

2 Always treat the casualty where you find him unless he is in any danger. If he has to be moved, temporarily immobilise the part as above.

3 If the ambulance is on the way, make the casualty as comfortable as possible without moving him. Place blankets, rolled coats and/or pillows alongside the injured area to keep it still and wait for the ambulance.

4 If there will be a long delay, immobilise the joints above and below the injury with padding and bandages using a sound part of the body as a splint.

5 While you are waiting for the ambulance, treat as on page 71 to prevent *Shock*.

BROKEN BONES (continued)

BROKEN LEG

Symptoms and signs
- Pain at the site of injury.
- Injured limb may look shorter than the other one.

If the thighbone is broken:
- The foot and knee may have fallen sideways.
- The thigh may look bent.

If the leg is broken below the knee:
- Probable open wound if the shin bone is broken.
- Foot fallen to one side although the knee is straight.

WHAT TO DO

1 If the ambulance is on the way and there is no immediate danger, do not move the casualty. Place one hand above and one hand below the injury to support it and place rolled coats, blankets and/ or cushions around the casualty's legs.

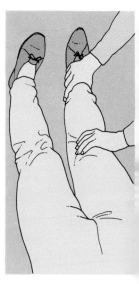

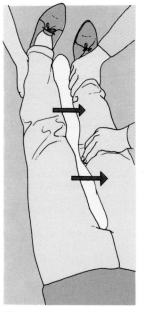

2 If the ambulance is delayed or the casualty has to be moved, immobilise the leg. Place soft padding between the knees and ankles and extra padding in the hollows above and below the knees and ankles.

3 Carefully bring the sound leg to the injured leg, *see left*.

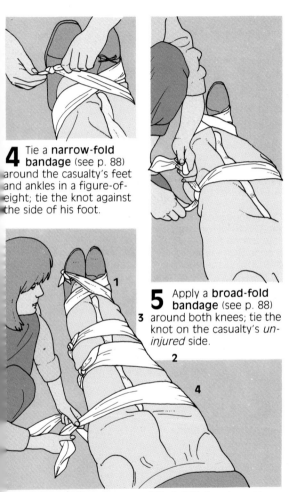

4 Tie a **narrow-fold bandage** (see p. 88) around the casualty's feet and ankles in a figure-of-eight; tie the knot against the side of his foot.

5 Apply a **broad-fold bandage** (see p. 88) around both knees; tie the knot on the casualty's *un-injured* side.

6 If there is time or there is a long journey ahead, add two more broad-fold bandages; one around the lower leg and one around the thighs. Avoid the site of the break; tie all knots on the un-injured side.

7 A fifth bandage may be added immediately below the site of the break if there is room.

BROKEN BONES *(continued)*

BROKEN PELVIS

Symptoms and signs

● Inability to move the lower part of the body without extreme pain; the pelvic area will be very tender.
● Casualty will be unable to stand up.
If there are internal injuries:
● Urine passed by the casualty may be blood-stained.
● Signs of *Internal bleeding* and *Shock* (see p. 70).

WHAT TO DO

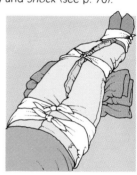

1 Lay the casualty down with legs straight or slightly bent with a coat under the knees – whichever is more comfortable.

2 Immobilise the casualty by passing **broad-fold bandages** (see p. 88) around the hips and pelvis, overlapping them by half; tie the knots in the centre.

3 Place padding between the ankles and the knees and tie a **narrow-fold bandage** (see p. 88) around the feet and ankles in a figure-of-eight and another **broad-fold bandage** around the knees.

4 Treat the casualty as described on page 71 to prevent *Shock* and wait for the ambulance.

BROKEN RIB

Symptoms and signs

● Sharp pain in affected side worsened by taking deep breaths or coughing.
● Casualty may hear crackling sound in chest.

WHAT TO DO

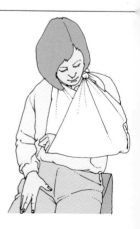

1 Sit the casualty down and support the arm on the injured side with an **arm sling** (see p. 92).

2 Take the casualty to hospital.

BROKEN COLLAR BONE

Symptoms and signs

● Casualty will probably be supporting the forearm on the injured side and inclining his head towards the injured side to relieve the pain.
● Reluctance to move arm on the injured side.
● Swelling or deformity visible at site of injury.

WHAT TO DO

1 Help the casualty support the arm on the injured side. Position it so that the fingers almost touch the opposite shoulder.

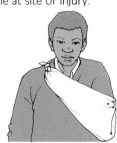

2 Place padding between the arm and the chest and support it with an **elevation sling** (see p. 93); take the casualty to hospital.

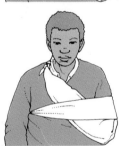

3 For extra support you can tie a **broad-fold bandage** (see p. 88) over the arm and right round the body.

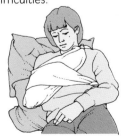

Treating serious rib injury

Rib injuries involving internal damage are serious. There may be breathing difficulties.

What to do

Support the casualty in a half-sitting position leaning towards the *injured* side. Place her arm in an **elevation sling** (see p. 93) and apply a **broad-fold bandage** (see p. 88).

BROKEN BONES *(continued)*

BROKEN ARM

Symptoms and signs

● Pain and tenderness at site of injury.
● Casualty will probably be supporting the hand, fore-arm and elbow of the injured arm.
● Inability to bend the arm if the bones are damaged at the elbow (see opposite).

WHAT TO DO

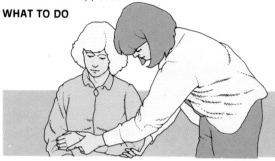

1 Gently bend the casualty's arm at the elbow and place it across her chest.

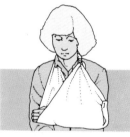

2 Place soft padding between the site of the injury and the body and support the arm with an **arm sling** (see p. 92).

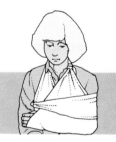

3 For extra support tie a **broad-fold bandage** (see p. 88) around the arm and trunk – avoid the site of the injury.

4 Take the casualty to hospital.

IMPORTANT

Do not bend the arm forcibly.

If the arm cannot be bent

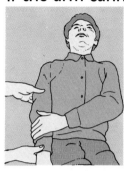

1 Help the casualty to lie down with his arm by his side or wherever he finds it most comfortable. Place padding between the arm and the chest.

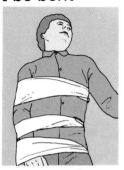

2 Carefully place three **broad-fold bandages** (see p. 88) around his arm and his body – avoid the site of injury. Await the ambulance.

BROKEN HAND OR FINGERS

Symptoms and signs

- Pain at site of injury.
- Possible deformity; fingers may be dislocated.
- Probable wound at site of break.

WHAT TO DO

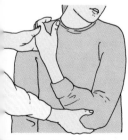

1 Raise the injured hand. Cover any wound with a **sterile dressing** (see p. 85).

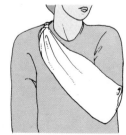

2 Place the hand in soft padding, support the arm in an **elevation sling** (see p. 93) and take the casualty to hospital.

B

BURNS

A burn is an injury caused by heat. Like any other wound, it breaks the skin and allows germs to enter, resulting in infection. In addition, fluid weeps into and out of the body tissues. This loss of fluid depletes the fluid part of the blood (*plasma*) and if a large area of the body is burnt there is a danger of *Shock* developing (see p. 70). A scald is an identical injury caused by contact with wet heat. All burns and scalds should be seen by a doctor or nurse as soon as possible.

Severe burns

If a large area of the casualty's body is burnt, lay him or her down, protecting the burnt surface from contact with the ground and treat for *Shock* (see p. 70). Do not give the casualty anything to eat or drink because he or she may need to have an anaesthetic later.

Symptoms and signs

● Extreme pain at the site of injury – although deep burns are sometimes less painful because the nerve endings may be destroyed.
● Swelling develops rapidly in the burnt area.
● Redness around the burn.
● Small bubbles of fluid (blisters) may develop under the top layer of skin at the point of contact with heat.
● Symptoms and signs of *Shock* (see p. 70).

WHAT TO DO

1 Remove the casualty from any danger *without endangering yourself* (see p. 11).

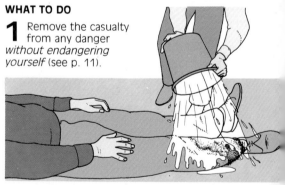

2 If the casualty's clothes are on fire, douse the flames with water or lay him down and smother the flames with a blanket or coat made of a non-flammable material. Do not let him rush outside.

IMPORTANT

● Never try to remove anything that is sticking to a burn.
● Never put any fats or ointments on a burn.
● Never put cotton wool on a burn.
● Never use an adhesive dressing.
● If there is no clean water available, use any cold, harmless liquid such as milk instead.

3 Hold the burnt part under cold running water for 10–20 minutes. If there is no running water, immerse the injured part in a bucket of CLEAN, cold water.

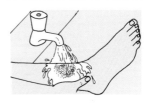

4 At the same time quickly but carefully remove any rings, watches or tight clothing from the injured area BEFORE it starts to swell.

5 Remove or cut away any clothing that has been soaked in a chemical (see overleaf) or boiling fluid; make sure that you do not injure yourself.

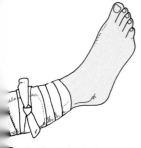
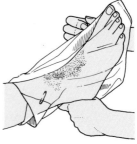

6 Protect the injury with a **sterile dressing** (see p. 85) large enough to cover the area completely.

7 If no dressing is available, cover the burn with a piece of CLEAN, non-fluffy material, or place a CLEAN polythene bag over a hand or foot.

8 Treat as on page 71 to prevent *Shock* developing and wait for the ambulance.

45

BURNS *(continued)*

SCALDED MOUTH AND THROAT

The mouth, throat and gut are lined with a very thin layer of skin called a mucous membrane. This membrane is easily damaged by drinking very hot fluid, swallowing chemicals that burn or by inhaling steam, and it swells up very quickly. Severe swelling in the mouth and throat can block the casualty's airway and prevent breathing (see p. 20).

Symptoms and signs

● Mouth and throat will be very painful and swollen.
● There may be difficulty in breathing.
● Skin around the casualty's mouth may appear red and blistered.
● If severe, symptoms and signs of *Shock* (see p. 70).

WHAT TO DO

1 Reassure the casualty

2 If she is conscious, wash her mouth out with cold water to cool the tissues, then give her frequent *sips* of cold water.

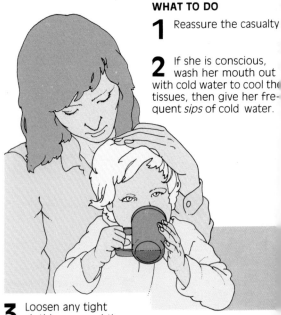

3 Loosen any tight clothing around the casualty's neck and chest.

4 Get the casualty to hospital as soon as possible.

5 If the casualty is unconscious, place her in the **recovery position** (see p. 22) treat as described on page 76.

CHEMICAL BURNS

Contact with some household cleaning materials, such as caustic soda and bleaches, or workshop materials such as paint stripper, can seriously damage the skin. You must act quickly to wash the chemicals off. If the eye is damaged, the treatment is the same but make sure that the contaminated water does not run down the face.

IMPORTANT

● Protect your hands and eyes from any contact with the chemical.
● Make sure the contaminated water drains away freely and safely.

Symptoms and signs

● Skin may be stained and there may be blisters at point of contact.
● Skin may be stinging.
● Redness around site of contact with chemical.

WHAT TO DO

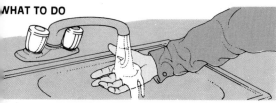

1 Flood the area by holding the injured part under cold running water for at least 10 minutes.

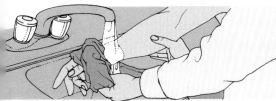

2 Remove any contaminated clothing from the casualty while you are flooding the area with cold water.

3 Continue treatment described on page 44 for burns.

C

CHOKING

This is the result of a blockage in the windpipe (airway). It can occur if food goes "down the wrong way" or if something like chewing gum, a boiled sweet, broken tooth or denture slips down the back of the throat.

Symptoms and signs

● Casualty suddenly brings her hand to her throat and is unable to speak.
● If not relieved, the casualty may turn blue in the face and the veins in the face and neck begin to stand out.
● If the blockage is still not removed, the casualty will lose consciousness.

WHAT TO DO

1 Ask the casualty if she can cough; if she can, encourage her to do so and *do not interfere*.

2 If she cannot cough, give her four sharp slaps (back slaps) between her shoulder blades with the heel of your hand.

3 If the back slaps do not work while the casualty is sitting or standing, help her to bend forward so that her head is lower than her chest and give her four more back slaps as above.

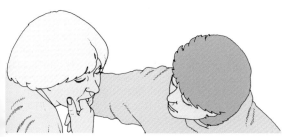

4 Check inside the casualty's mouth. Tell the casualty to run her finger around the back of her mouth and try to hook out any foreign mater she finds. Be prepared to do it yourself.

5 If the casualty loses consciousness, **open and clear the airway** (see pp. 20–1) and begin **mouth-to-mouth** if necessary (see p. 24).

Choking in babies and small children

If the casualty is a baby or small child, follow the same procedure but use less force when applying the back slaps, see below.

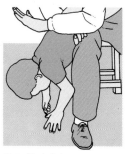

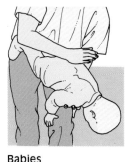

Small children
Lay the child across your thigh with his head down below his chest and give four quick slaps between the shoulders.

Babies
Lay the baby along your forearm so that she is face down and her head is below her chest. Support her head and shoulders with one hand and give four light slaps between the shoulders with the other hand.

C

CONVULSIONS IN YOUNG CHILDREN

Most common in children between the ages of one and four, convulsions are generally caused by a very high temperature (fever), serious tummy upset, fright or temper. Although they appear alarming, particularly if the child is holding his or her breath, they are not dangerous.

Symptoms and signs

● Child may be flushed and sweating with a very hot forehead.
● Child's muscles may stiffen and his back may be arched; she may begin jerking movements (convulsions).
● The eyes may be rolled upwards.
● Child's face may appear blue if he is breath-holding.

WHAT TO DO

1 Loosen any clothing around the child's neck and chest.

2 If convulsions are severe, clear a space around him to prevent him injuring himself.

3 Wipe any froth from around his mouth.

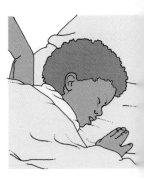

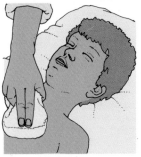

5 When convulsions stop, place the child in the **recovery position** (see p. 22) and cover him with LIGHT bedclothes such as a sheet.

6 Reassure the child and seek medical aid.

4 Cool him by removing his clothes and any bedclothes and sponging him with tepid water; work from the head down.

CRAMP

This is a sudden pain in a limb caused by a tightening, or contraction, of a muscle or group of muscles. Cramp, particularly in the calf muscles, often occurs in the middle of the night. It can normally be relieved by stretching the affected muscles as shown below.

A person who has been sweating heavily may develop cramp. To relieve this, give the casualty a tumbler of water containing a teaspoon of salt.

WHAT TO DO

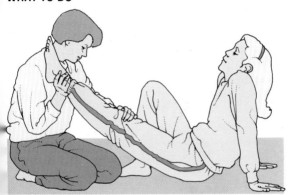

For cramp in the thigh
Straighten the casualty's leg and gently but firmly press the knee down and pull the lower part of the leg up and forward to stretch the muscles.

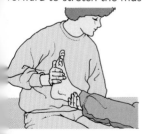

For cramp in the calf
Straighten the casualty's knee and push her foot up as far as it will go.

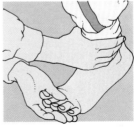

For cramp in the foot
Straighten the casualty's bent toes by pushing them upwards and help her to stand on the ball of her foot.

D

DISLOCATED JOINT

This is the displacement of bones at a joint – the point where two or more bones meet. Joints are held together by tough bands of fibre called *ligaments*. Dislocation occurs if there is a particularly violent or sudden twisting strain on the joint which tears the ligament. It is extremely painful and, in some cases, it may be difficult to distinguish between a dislocated joint and a broken bone. If in doubt, always treat the injury as a broken bone (see pp. 37–43).

Symptoms and signs

- Extreme pain around the affected joint.
- Inability to move the affected part.
- Swelling, often severe, around the injured joint.
- Severe deformity at site of injury.

WHAT TO DO

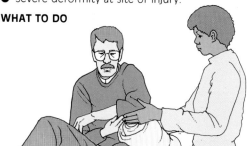

1 Help the casualty into the position he finds most comfortable.

2 Support the injured part with pillows, rolled blankets and/or bandages and slings as applicable.

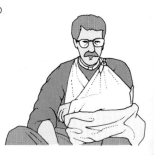

3 Await the arrival of medical aid.

IMPORTANT

- Move the affected limb as little as possible.
- Never try to manipulate a dislocated joint – you will worsen the injury.

ELECTRICAL INJURY

An electric current passed through the body can cause serious burns at the point of entry and exit. Although these burns look small, they are likely to be deep. In addition, the electric current can cause quivering of the heart muscle or it can stop the heart, in which case breathing will stop.

Causes of electrical injury

Any low-voltage appliance used in the home or workshop, such as food mixers or drills, can cause electrical injury if not correctly wired or insulated. Young children are at risk because they often try to play with wires, plugs or sockets.

Whatever the cause of the injury you must *never* touch the casualty with your bare hands until you are sure that the current has been broken and you are not in any danger (see p. 10).

Symptoms and signs

● Deep burns at point of entry and exit of electricity.
● Possible unconsciousness.
● Symptoms and signs of *Shock* (see p. 70).
● Lack of breathing and heartbeat – casualty may look grey (ashen) if both stopped at once.

WHAT TO DO

1 Break the current if possible by switching it off at the mains or knocking the casualty's limb clear of the contact with a non-conducting implement (see p. 10). Seek medical aid.

2 If the casualty is unconscious, **check breathing** (see p. 18). If it has stopped, begin **mouth-to-mouth** and, if necessary, **chest compression** (see pp. 24–7).

3 If the casualty is unconscious but breathing, place him in the **recovery position** (see p. 22) and treat as described on page 76.

4 Treat any burns as described on pages 44–7.

5 While waiting for the ambulance, treat as described on page 71 to prevent *Shock*.

EPILEPSY

This is a tendency towards fits or seizures caused by a brief disruption in the electrical activity of the brain. There are two main types of fit – major fits (see below and opposite) and minor fits. Minor fits often pass unnoticed. If you see someone having a major fit, do not be frightened. Follow the steps described on these two pages. Let the fit run its course and do not interfere.

Symptoms and signs

These generally follow a set pattern:

● Sudden collapse; the casualty may let out a strange cry as he falls.

● Muscles stiffen then relax, then begin jerking movements (convulsions) – these may be violent.

● Froth may appear around the casualty's mouth – this may be blood-stained if the casualty has bitten his tongue or the inside of his mouth.

● After the fit is over, usually five minutes at the most, the casualty will regain consciousness but may be dazed and confused. This can last up to an hour and he may want to sleep.

WHAT TO DO

1 Keep calm and stop anyone interfering with the casualty.

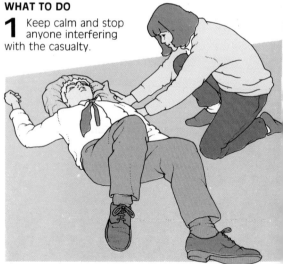

2 Clear a space around him so that he does not hurt himself or move him out of the way of traffic. If possible put something soft *around* his head.

IMPORTANT

● Never try to hold a person down.
● Never put anything in the casualty's mouth
– especially not your fingers.
● Never give a person anything to eat or drink during a fit.
● There is no need to call an ambulance unless one fit follows another without the person regaining consciousness in between.

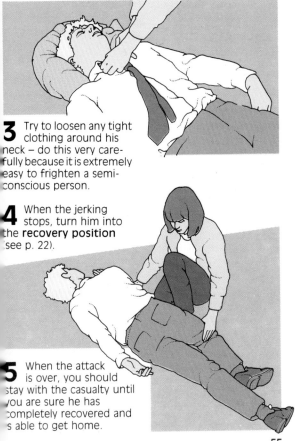

3 Try to loosen any tight clothing around his neck – do this very carefully because it is extremely easy to frighten a semi-conscious person.

4 When the jerking stops, turn him into the **recovery position** (see p. 22).

5 When the attack is over, you should stay with the casualty until you are sure he has completely recovered and is able to get home.

E

EYE INJURY

Small foreign bodies such as splinters of metal, glass or wood scratching the surface of a person's eye or becoming embedded in the eye are the most common cause of eye injury. Examine the eye as described below, but if in doubt, cover the eye with a sterile dressing and seek medical aid.

IMPORTANT

Never try to remove anything that is on the coloured part of the eye or embedded in the eye; cover the eye with a dressing and seek medical aid immediately.

Symptoms and signs

● Pain in the affected eye.

WHAT TO DO

1 Tell the casualty not to rub her eye. Ask her to sit down in a chair facing a light. Wash your hands.

2 Ask the the casualty to look up. Support her chin with one hand and gently draw the lower eyelid down and outward with the other hand.

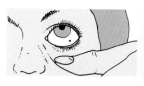

3 If you can see the object on the white part of the eye or the eyelid, lift it off with a moistened wisp of cotton wool or corner of a clean tissue.

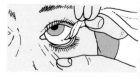

4 If you think the particle is on the upper lid, ask the casualty to look down. Grasp the upper lid and draw it down and out over the lower lid.

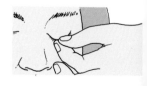

5 If you are not successful, help her to put her eye under water and tell her to blink; the particle should float off.

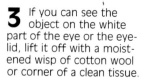

6 If you cannot remove the particle, cover the eye with a **sterile dressing** (see p. 85) and seek medical aid.

FAINTING

This is a brief period of unconsciousness which happens when the flow of blood to the brain is temporarily reduced. It is sometimes known as "nervous shock" because it can be brought on by pain or emotion. It can also occur if a person has to stand still for a long time in a warm atmosphere; moving the feet and/or changing position can help prevent this. If the casualty lies down with his or her legs raised above chest (heart) level, recovery will normally be quick and complete.

Symptoms and signs

● Casualty will feel weak, faint and giddy.
● Skin will be very pale.
● Pulse will be very SLOW.

WHAT TO DO

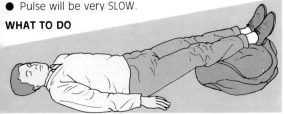

1 Help the casualty to lie down and raise his feet above the level of his chest.

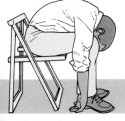

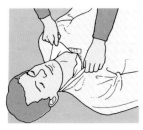

2 If there is no room to lie down, help him to lean forward with his head between his knees.

3 Loosen any tight clothing around his neck, chest and waist.

4 Make sure the casualty has enough air. Open the window and/or ask people not to crowd round him; fan his face if necessary.

5 If you are in any doubt about his condition, seek medical aid.

F

FOREIGN BODIES

Children in particular have a habit of putting small objects in their noses, ears or mouths.

If a child has swallowed something, he or she could choke; treat as described on page 48. If someone swallows a fishbone, *do not try to remove it*. Reassure him or her and seek medical aid as soon as possible.

FOREIGN BODY IN THE EAR
WHAT TO DO

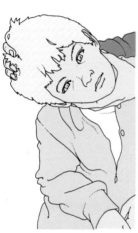

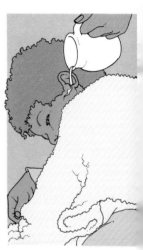

1 If the casualty has pushed something into his ear, tilt the head so that the affected ear is downward; the object may drop out.

2 If there is an insect in the casualty's ear, help him to lie down with the affected ear up. Gently pour clean tepid water into the ear; the insect may float to the surface.

3 If the object or insect does not come out easily, seek medical aid as soon as possible.

FOREIGN BODY IN THE NOSE
WHAT TO DO

1 Reassure the casualty. Tell him to breathe through his mouth.

2 Take him to hospital as quickly as possible

58

FROSTBITE

Frostbite, that is, freezing of the skin and underlying tissues, is a serious condition. It can occur if parts of the body, generally the extremities such as the fingers, toes, nose and ears, are exposed to prolonged or intense cold. Permanent damage can result if it is not treated promptly. However, Frostbite can be accompanied by *Hypothermia* (see p. 64) – the latter MUST be treated first.

Symptoms and signs

Prickling sensation in affected area followed by gradual loss of feeling.

Skin in affected area will feel hard and cold.

Skin will become mottled blue or even white.

IMPORTANT

● Do not warm the affected area with direct heat (for example, a hot-water bottle or electric blanket).
● Do not allow the casualty to walk on a frost-bitten foot.
● Do not rub the affected area.

WHAT TO DO

1 Examine the casualty for signs of *Hypothermia* (see p. 64).

2 Remove any tight clothing or jewellery from the affected area.

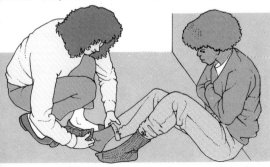

3 Cover the affected area with warm, dry clothes. The casualty can put frostbitten hands in her armpits.

4 Place a soft dressing over the affected area and seek medical aid as soon as possible.

HEAD INJURIES

The movement and functions of the body are controlled by the *nervous system* – the brain, spinal cord and nerves. The brain is a very delicate structure which acts like a central exchange and controls the rest of the system. It is surrounded and protected by the skull.

What can go wrong
A blow to the head can cause bruising (bleeding under the skin) or it can cut the scalp (the skin around the skull) but it can also damage the skull. Moreover, whether or not the skull is fractured, the blow can also cause a condition of unconsciousness known as *concussion*. This is caused by a temporary shake-up of the brain – rather like jelly wobbling against the side of a jelly mould.

Why a head injury is serious
Any person with a head injury MUST be seen by a doctor as soon as possible because there may be delayed effects such as swelling of the brain, or bleeding into the brain or the area between the brain and the skull, which causes unconsciousness to deepen.

Symptoms and signs
● Bleeding from the scalp.
Of concussion:
● A period of unconsciousness – although this may be so short that neither you nor the casualty is aware of it.
● Casualty may be dazed and confused.
● Casualty may not remember the incident or anything that happened immediately beforehand.
Of skull fracture:
● Blood, or blood-stained fluid, coming from inside the casualty's ear or nose.
● Discoloration around the eyelids (black eye) or on the white part of the eye.
Danger signs:
● Deep unconsciousness, *coma* (see p. 76).
● Casualty making snoring sounds as she breathes.
● The pupils of the eyes may be abnormally small, large or of different sizes.
● Unusually slow pulse.

WHAT TO DO

1 If the casualty does not appear to be seriously injured, advise her to see a doctor at a hospital or surgery, as soon as possible.

2 If the casualty was unconscious, even for a short time, arrange for her to be taken to hospital immediately by ambulance.

3 If the casualty is unconscious, treat as described on page 76. Remember that you must maintain an open airway, breathing and circulation.

4 Treat any *Wounds* or *Broken bones* (see pp. 78–82 and 37–43).

Treating a scalp wound

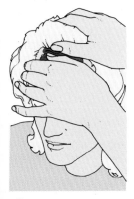 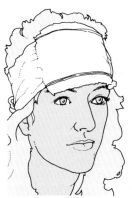

1 Control bleeding by pressing the edges of the wound together with your thumbs as shown.

2 Place a **sterile dressing** (see p. 84) over the wound and secure it with the attached bandage.

3 Help the casualty to sit down on the ground leaning against a wall. Support her head and shoulders with cushions.

4 If the casualty is unconscious, place her in the **recovery position** (see p. 22).

H

HEART ATTACK

The heart muscle needs oxygen and this is supplied by the blood vessels of the heart – the coronary arteries.

Causes and types of heart attack

There are several varieties and causes of heart attack. Firstly, because of the effects of disease of the heart or lungs, the heart muscle may become progressively weaker over a period of time and may fail. The casualty will be increasingly breathless and his skin will look blue.

Sometimes, the coronary arteries become narrowed, causing "crushing" chest pain after moderately severe exercise. This is called *angina*.

Complete blockage of the coronary arteries – *coronary thrombosis* – can also occur. The resulting pain is similar to that of *angina* but may be more severe. (It may be difficult to tell the difference between the two types of pain.)

Coronary thrombosis can stop the heart altogether. You will not be able to feel a pulse (see p. 19); this is called *cardiac arrest*. The casualty will lose consciousness rapidly because there is no blood supply to the brain and breathing will stop.

Symptoms and signs

● Sudden increasing breathlessness.
● Casualty's skin may look blue.
Signs of angina:
● Casualty complains of severe crushing pain in his chest – particularly in the left side – which radiates out towards his arms and up to his neck.
● Pulse may be irregular.
● Skin will be pale or ashen.
Signs of coronary thrombosis:
● Any of the above symptoms and signs.
● Possible unconsciousness.
Signs of cardiac arrest:
● Lack of heartbeat and breathing.

Cardiac arrest

If the casualty's heart has stopped beating, lay him flat on his back on a firm surface and begin **mouth-to-mouth** (see p. 24) and **chest compression** (see p. 26) *immediately*.

WHAT TO DO

1 If the casualty appears breath-less and is complaining of severe chest pain, sit him down in a chair or on the floor leaning up against a wall, whichever is nearer.

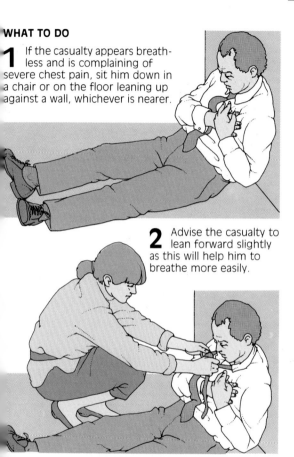

2 Advise the casualty to lean forward slightly as this will help him to breathe more easily.

3 Loosen any tight clothing around his neck, chest and waist.

4 Ask the casualty's if he is carrying any drugs speci-fically for a heart condition. If he is, administer them as prescribed.

5 If there is no improvement after five minutes at the most, or the casualty has no history of heart problems, call an ambulance immediately.

6 If the casualty becomes *unconscious*, treat as des-cribed on page 76 while waiting for the ambulance.

H

HYPOTHERMIA

This is a condition that develops when the body temperature drops below 35°C (95°F). It is most likely to occur when the weather is very cold.

Hypothermia in the home
Elderly people and young children are very susceptible to chilling. The elderly and babies can lose a dangerous amount of body heat in conditions that may not appear to be particularly cold, such as sitting in a poorly heated house. This is more common with old people, especially if they are living on their own, because they may not use enough bedding, their diet may be inadequate or they may try to save money by not lighting a fire or turning on a heater.

Symptoms and signs
● Casualty's movements may be clumsy and his speech may be slurred.
● Casualty will slow down both physically and mentally and may become very irritable.
● The skin will feel very cold.
● Casualty may be pale and shivering badly.
● If hypothermia is not treated quickly, the casualty will lose consciousness.
Hypothermia in babies:
● The baby will be very drowsy and floppy.
● Baby's face, hands and feet will feel very cold but they may look bright pink and healthy.

Treating babies

Hypothermia in babies is a dangerous condition and you should seek medical aid immediately. Treat as described below while you are waiting.

What you can do
While you are waiting for medical aid, take the baby into a sleeping bag or your bed with you to rewarm her gradually with body heat. A small baby can be put down the front of your shirt.

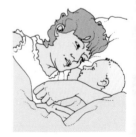

IMPORTANT

● Do not let the casualty walk about or rub his or her skin to warm up.
● Warm a casualty gradually – never use a hot-water bottle or electric blanket.
● Do not give the casualty any alcohol.

WHAT TO DO

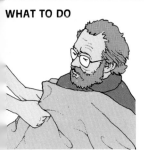

1 Warm the casualty gradually. Wrap him in a blanket and warm the room, or carry him to warmer surroundings.

2 If the casualty has been outside in wet clothes, bring him into warm surroundings and give him some dry clothes to put on.

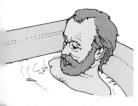

3 A *healthy* adult can be rewarmed more rapidly in a warm bath; the bath should feel warm but *not* hot against the back of your hand.

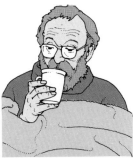

4 Give the casualty sips of a warm (*not hot*) drink; be prepared to hold the mug for him.

5 Encourage the casualty to move his limbs to improve circulation but *do not rub the skin*.

6 If the casualty is unconscious, place him in the **recovery position** (see p. 22), and keep **checking breathing** (see p. 18) and **circulation** (see p. 19) until the doctor or ambulance arrives.

MUSCLE INJURY

Muscles move bones at the joints. Most *muscles* consist of a fleshy part that is joined directly to a bone at one end. The other end tapers and ends in a fibrous *tendon* which is attached to another bone. Movement occurs when a muscle contracts and pulls one bone towards another.

Muscles and their tendons can be strained or torn by a sudden contraction or awkward movement. This is commonly known as a "strained muscle" or "pulled muscle".

Symptoms and signs

● Pain in the affected area, particularly if the casualty tries to repeat the movement that caused the injury.
● Stiffness in the affected area; this will normally develop gradually.
● Swelling and discoloration around the site of injury.

WHAT TO DO

1 Help the casualty into a comfortable position supporting the injured part by hand.

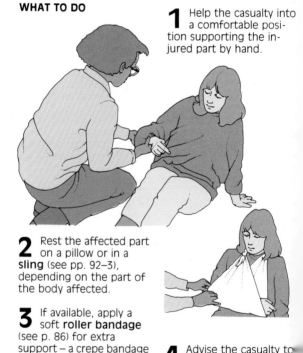

2 Rest the affected part on a pillow or in a **sling** (see pp. 92–3), depending on the part of the body affected.

3 If available, apply a soft **roller bandage** (see p. 86) for extra support – a crepe bandage is ideal.

4 Advise the casualty to see a doctor.

NOSE-BLEED

Nose-bleeds are normally caused by a blow to the nose or, in some cases, a violent sneeze or by blowing the nose too hard. Sometimes there may be no apparent cause.

IMPORTANT

If a nose-bleed follows a blow to a person's head, he or she could have a fractured skull (see *Head injury*, p. 60).

WHAT TO DO

1 Help the casualty to sit down and tell him to lean forward, pinch the soft part of his nose and breathe through his mouth. He may need to do this for 10–20 minutes; be prepared to help him.

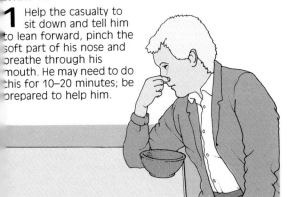

2 Give the casualty a bowl and tell him to spit out any fluid in his mouth; swallowing can disturb the blood clot and the blood may make him feel sick.

3 When the bleeding stops, advise the casualty NOT to blow his nose for some hours because it may restart the bleeding.

4 If the bleeding does not stop after 20 minutes, call a doctor immediately.

P

POISONING

Poisons are substances that result in temporary or permanent damage to the body if taken in sufficient quantities. They can be taken into the body in several different ways: by being swallowed (for example, pills or poisonous berries); by being breathed in (inhaled); by being injected under the skin (for example, by hypodermic syringe, animal or insect bites); by absorption through the skin (for example, agricultural or garden weedkillers or some insecticides).

Symptoms and signs

● Casualty may be very drowsy or even unconscious; this will depend on the poison and quantity taken.
● Container known to have had a poisonous substance in it, loose tablets or poisonous plant near the casualty.
● Burns around the lips if the casualty has taken a corrosive poison.
● Possible vomiting, or even diarrhoea at a later stage.
● Possible convulsions.

IMPORTANT

● Do not leave the casualty alone.
● If a person has swallowed a corrosive poison (e.g., bleach or disinfectant), never try to make him or her sick; anything that burns going down the gullet will burn coming up.
● Keep poisons locked away and out of reach of children.
● Keep children away from poisonous plants or plants with poisonous berries.

Poisonous plants

Some plants can be dangerous if eaten. Children are often attracted by the bright berries of these plants and may eat them. Many houseplants are also poisonous so keep them out of reach of children.

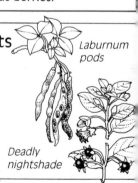

Laburnum pods

Deadly nightshade

WHAT TO DO

1 If the casualty is conscious, quickly ask her what she has taken and how much because she may lose consciousness at any time.

2 Call the doctor or ambulance. Tell them what you think the casualty has taken; the person taking the call may tell you what to do while you are waiting for medical aid.

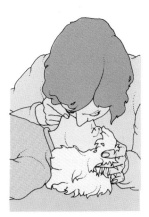

4 If **mouth-to-mouth** is necessary, be careful not to get any of the poison on your mouth. If possible wash the poison off the face and use **mouth-to-nose** (see pp. 24–5 and 28–9).

5 If you are certain that the casualty has NOT taken a corrosive poison, but has *only* taken tablets or berries, it may help to make her sick by putting a finger down the back of her throat.

6 Transfer the casualty to hospital as soon as possible with any pills, medicines, empty containers or poisonous leaves and/or berries found near her and any sample of vomit.

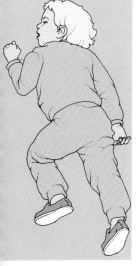

3 If the casualty is unconscious but breathing, turn her into the **recovery position** (see p. 2) and treat as described on page 76 for *Unconsciousness*.

SHOCK

This is a condition in which the blood circulation, which supplies oxygen to the tissues, fails. There are many possible causes and they fall into two main categories. Firstly, the amount of blood circulating in the body may become reduced so that there is not enough left to supply all the body cells with oxygen. Secondly, the heart may become weak, so the pressure of the circulating blood falls, or the heart may stop. Vital brain cells can die after only three minutes without oxygen.

What causes shock
It can be the result of bleeding – external (see p. 30) or internal (see below); heart attacks (see p. 62); or loss of body fluids following widespread burns (see p. 44), severe allergic reaction (see p. 74), serious vomiting or diarrhoea.

Symptoms and signs
● Skin becomes very pale and grey; this is most obvious inside the lips or under fingernails.
● Skin will be cold and moist with sweat.
● Pulse will be rapid but weak (see p. 19).
● Breathing will be shallow and fast.
● Casualty will become restless and may begin yawning.
● Casualty may complain that she is very thirsty.
● Finally, she may lose consciousness and die if treatment is not successful.

Internal bleeding

This can be the result of damage to an internal organ; a penetrating wound; an illness that causes sudden, severe bleeding within the body cavity; or an injury that causes a large bone such as the thighbone or pelvis to break. Treat as described for *Shock* (opposite) if you notice *any* of the symptoms and signs below.

Symptoms and signs
● Any of the symptoms and signs of *Shock* developing rapidly; there may be no visible injury.
● Casualty may be unnaturally quiet.
● Casualty may, however, complain of pain, sometimes severe, in the chest or abdomen.
● An unusually large amount of swelling around the injured part.

IMPORTANT

● Do not give the casualty anything to eat or drink; he or she may need an anaesthetic later.
● Never use a hot-water bottle or electric blanket to warm the casualty.

WHAT TO DO

1 Stop external bleeding as soon as possible using **direct pressure** and **elevation** (see p. 30).

2 Reassure the casualty and move her as little as possible.

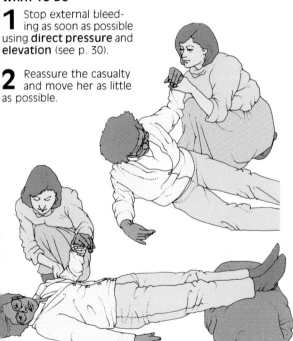

3 Lay the casualty down. Raise her feet by putting a cushion underneath them and turn her head to one side.

4 Keep the casualty comfortable, for example, wrap her in a blanket if it is cold.

5 Wait for the ambulance to arrive.

6 If the casualty is unconscious, treat as described on p. 76.

SPLINTERS

Small pieces of wood, metal or glass can easily become embedded in the skin. Splinters need to be removed because they are dirty and if left in the skin may cause infection.

Normally, splinters are easy to remove (see below). If, however, the end is not visible, let a doctor or nurse remove it because it is easy to push the splinter further in or break it, making it more difficult to remove later.

IMPORTANT

● Never dig into the skin to remove a splinter.
● Always keep your tetanus inoculations up-to-date.

WHAT TO DO

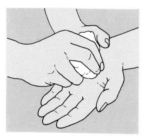

1 Clean the area around the splinter with soap and water (see p. 72).

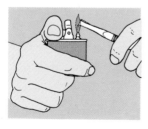

2 Sterilise a pair of tweezers by passing them through the flame from a match or lighter.

3 Allow the tweezers to cool. Do not wipe the soot off or touch the ends.

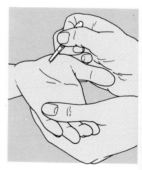

4 Holding the tweezers as near to the skin as possible, grasp the end of the splinter. Gently pull the splinter out in the opposite direction to that in which it entered the skin.

5 If the splinter breaks, do not continue, seek medical aid.

SPRAINED JOINT

This occurs when the ligaments that hold bones
together at a joint are over-stretched or torn. A
broken bone may be mistaken for a sprain. If in
doubt, treat as a broken bone (see pp. 37–43).

Symptoms and signs

- Severe pain at the injured joint.
- Bruising and discoloration around the injured area.
- The joint will swell; this may be gradual.
- The casualty may not be able to move the joint, or
stand up if a knee or ankle is affected.

WHAT TO DO

1 Help the casualty into
the position she finds
most comfortable and
raise the injured part.

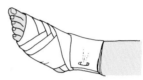

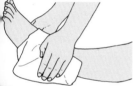

2 If the sprain is recent,
place a **cold com-
press** on the joint; leave it
for 30 minutes. This slows
down the blood flow to
the area, minimising swelling and reducing pain.

3 Cover the area with a
layer of cotton wool;
secure this with a **roller
bandage** (see p. 86).

4 If the injury is to the
wrist, elbow or
shoulder, support her in-
jured arm with an **arm
sling** (see p. 92).

5 Seek medical aid because the casualty
may need an X-ray.

Making cold compresses

You can do this in two ways: soak a piece of
material in cold water, wring it out and place it
over the injury (replace this type of pack every 10
minutes), or make an ice pack as shown below.

Making an ice pack
Fill a plastic bag ½–⅔
full of ice. Add a little
salt, squeeze the air out
of the bag and seal it.
Wrap it in a thin towel
and place it over the
injured area.

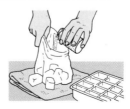

STINGS

Insects such as bees leave small stings embedded in the skin which should be removed. Wasp and hornet stings are more alarming than dangerous.

WHAT TO DO

1 If the sting is still in the skin, remove it with a pair of tweezers; sterilise them before you begin (see p. 72).

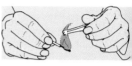

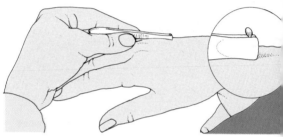

2 Hold the tweezers as close to the casualty's skin as possible. Grasp the barb of the sting with the tweezers and pull it out. Avoid the poison sac at the top of the sting; squeezing it will force more poison into the casualty's hand.

3 Apply a **cold compress** (see p. 73) to reduce pain and swelling, and rest the injured part.

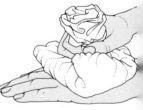

4 If you are in any doubt about the casualty, seek medical aid.

IMPORTANT

If a person is unduly sensitive to stings or is stung in the throat, the throat will swell very quickly and could block the airway and prevent breathing. Give him or her cold water to drink or ice to suck and seek medical aid immediately. If breathing becomes difficult or the casualty is unconscious, place him or her in the *recovery position* (see p. 22).

SUFFOCATION

This can occur when air is prevented from entering the mouth, nose or windpipe as, for instance, when someone is drowning or buried under a fall of earth or sand. It can also occur if a baby is lying face down on a pillow or a child pulls a polythene bag over his or her face.

Suffocation will also result when the air that enters the airway is polluted with smoke and poisonous fumes (see p. 11) or poisonous gas, for example, exhaust fumes from a petrol engine.

Symptoms and signs

● Difficulty in breathing; breathing may appear laboured and noisy.
● Frothing at the mouth.
● Lips and fingernails may become blue if the cause is not removed promptly.
● Possible unconsciousness.

WHAT TO DO

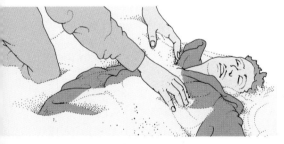

1 Remove the cause of the obstruction from the face and neck, or remove the casualty from the danger, *without endangering yourself*.

2 If the casualty is buried under a pile of earth or sand, try to remove it as far back as the hips so that his chest can expand during breathing.

3 **Open and clear the airway** (see pp. 20–21) and **check breathing** (see p. 18).

4 If the casualty does not begin breathing after the airway has been opened, begin **mouth-to-mouth** immediately (see p. 24).

5 Seek medical aid immediately; keep **checking breathing** while you wait for the ambulance.

U

UNCONSCIOUSNESS

This is a state in which a casualty becomes insensible because of an interruption in the normal function of his or her brain. Unconsciousness differs from sleep in that you cannot wake a person up by shouting at him or her or by using a painful stimulus such as a pinch. It may develop gradually or suddenly and it can be the result of injury or serious illness.

Why is unconsciousness dangerous?

The danger of unconsciousness is that the normal reflexes that allow you to breathe without choking while asleep may not work properly or even work at all (see p. 20).

Levels of unconsciousness

The casualty may pass through various levels of confusion and stupor (behaving rather like a drunk person) before becoming completely unconscious (coma) and will pass through the same stages in reverse as he or she recovers.

WHAT TO DO

1 Gently shake the casualty by the shoulders and ask her loudly if she is all right – give her 5–10 seconds to respond.

IMPORTANT

● Never leave an unconscious person alone.
● Do not give anyone who is, or who has been, unconscious *anything* to eat or drink.
● Anyone who has been unconscious, even for a short time, *must* be seen by a doctor as soon as possible.

2 If there is no response, look, listen and feel for **breathing** (see p. 18).

3 If she is not breathing, or she is making snoring or gurgling sounds, **open the airway** (see p. 20).

4 If the casualty is still not breathing, **clear the airway** (see p. 21).

5 If she is not breathing after the airway has been opened and cleared, begin **mouth-to-mouth** (see p. 24) and, if necessary, **chest compression** (see p. 26).

6 Very gently examine the casualty from head to foot and treat any injury you find.

7 Look out for any medical warning signs such as Medic-alert bracelets or information cards worn or carried by the casualty; they may indicate the cause of the casualty's condition.

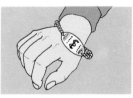

8 If the casualty is now breathing normally, place her in the **recovery position** (see p. 22) and await the ambulance.

9 Check **circulation** (see p. 19), **breathing** (see p. 18) and **level of consciousness** (see opposite) every few minutes; note any changes in the casualty's condition.

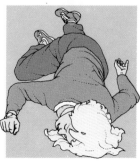

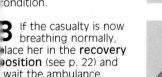

WOUNDS

A wound is an injury that breaks the skin or other tissues and that can allow blood to escape from the body and germs to enter it. First aid for wounds is described below and opposite. This treatment will have to be adapted for some injuries (see pp.80–2).

The priority is always to stop any external bleeding immediately, because if a large amount of blood is lost from the circulatory system, there will not be enough to circulate the oxygen to all the tissues and *Shock* (see p. 70), and eventually death, can result (see below and *Controlling severe bleeding*, p. 30).

Symptoms and signs

● Evidence of severe blood loss.
● Symptoms and signs of *Shock* (see p. 70) if blood loss is prolonged.

WHAT TO DO

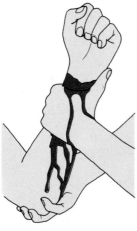

2 Help the casualty to lie down (see p. 30).

3 Place a **sterile dressing** (see p. 85) over the wound – it must be large enough to extend well beyond the area of the injury. If there is no dressing available, improvise (see p. 94).

4 If there is a foreign body in the wound, do not remove it; treat as described on page 82.

5 If blood begins to show through the first dressing, do not remove it; put more dressings on top.

6 While waiting for the ambulance, watch for symptoms and signs of *Shock* (see p. 70) and treat the casualty accordingly.

1 Raise the limb and apply **direct pressure** (see p.30) by pressing over the wound with your thumb and/or fingers as necessary. Use a pad if possible.

SMALL CUTS AND GRAZES

With small cuts and grazes, the bleeding will normally stop of its own accord. The aim of treatment is to clean and dress the wound as soon as possible to prevent germs entering the body.

You will need:
● A dressing (see p. 84).
● Soap and water.
● Cotton wool, gauze swabs or antiseptic wipes.

WHAT TO DO

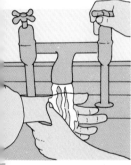

1 If the wound is dirty, rinse it under cold running water until clean.

2 Sit the casualty down and cover the wound temporarily with clean gauze or a tissue.

3 Collect all the equipment together and place it on a piece of clean paper towel.

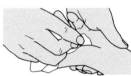

4 Gently clean around the wound with soap and water using the cotton wool, gauze swabs or antiseptic wipes. Work from the wound outward and use a fresh swab for each stroke.

5 Carefully remove any *loose* foreign matter such as glass, metal or gravel with clean cotton wool or gauze swabs or tweezers (see p. 72).

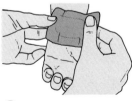

6 Dry the area and apply an **adhesive dressing** (see p. 84).

IMPORTANT

● Never dress a wound with cotton wool or anything fluffy.
● Never cough over the wound or equipment you are going to use.

WOUNDS *(continued)*

WOUND TO PALM OF HAND

This injury will bleed profusely and it may be
difficult to apply pressure in the normal way.
Bandage as described here but make sure there is
nothing embedded in the wound before you start.

WHAT TO DO

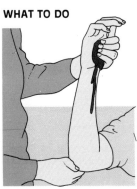

1 Sit or lay the casualty
down and raise his
hand above the level of
his chest (heart). Apply
direct pressure (see p. 30).
Use a pad if possible.

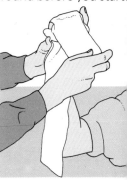

3 Leaving the short end
of the bandage free,
wrap the long part around
the fist so that it pulls the
fingers down over the pad.

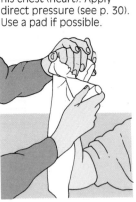

2 Cover the wound with
a **sterile dressing**
(see p. 85) and ask the
casualty to clench his fist
over the pad; he may need
some help.

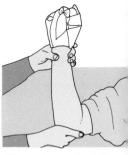

4 Tie the ends of the
bandage together
across the top of the casualty's knuckles using a **reef
knot** (see p. 89).

5 Support the arm in
an **elevation sling**
(see p. 93) and seek
medical aid.

BLEEDING FROM A TOOTH SOCKET

This can occur after the accidental loss of a tooth
or it could happen some while after a tooth has
been removed by a dentist.

WHAT TO DO

3 Tell the casualty to bite hard on the pad for 10–20 minutes.

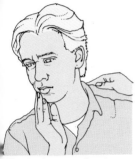

1 Sit the casualty down and ask him to incline his head towards the injured side.

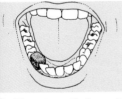

2 Place a small piece of tightly packed gauze in but not into the tooth socket; it must project above the level of the remaining teeth.

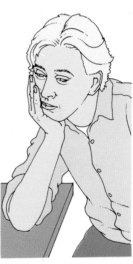

4 He may find it easier if he puts his elbow on a table and rests his jaw on his cupped hand.

5 Seek dental or medical aid as soon as you can.

Saving a tooth

If you find the displaced tooth near the casualty,
keep it safe because the dentist or doctor may be
able to replace it. *Do not wash it in water*. Place the
tooth in a clean container, mark the container
clearly and send or take it to the dentist or hospital
with the casualty.

81

WOUNDS *(continued)*

EMBEDDED OBJECTS IN WOUND

Do not remove any object that is embedded in a wound because it may be plugging the wound preventing bleeding and you may do more damage by pulling it out. Leave it well alone. Build up padding round the object and secure the padding with a bandage as described below.

WHAT TO DO

1 Help the casualty to lie down and raise the injured part.

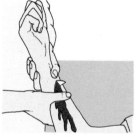

2 Control severe bleeding by pressing the area immediately above and below the object.

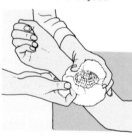

3 Drape a piece of gauze over the wound and the embedded object. Very carefully place pads of cotton wool around the object until they are at least the same height as the object.

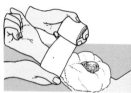

4 Place the end of a **roller bandage** (see p. 86) over the padding nearest you and make two straight turns.

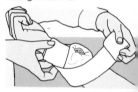

5 Pass the bandage under the limb and bring it up over the top edge of the padding.

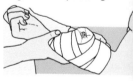

6 Continue making these diagonal turns above and below the padding until it is secure.

7 Immobilise the limb as for a broken bone (see pp. 37–43) and wait for the ambulance.

DRESSINGS AND BANDAGES

There are various dressings and bandages available. The type you use and the method of application will depend on the injury and the part of the body affected. Where possible, always use the correct dressing as shown on the following pages. However, if the right dressing is not available, improvise using any clean NON-FLUFFY material (see p. 94).

Applying dressings and bandages

It is very important to minimise the risk of infection. If you can, always wash your hands before you apply a dressing. Stand in front of the casualty on his or her injured side and keep the part to be bandaged supported until you are certain that the sling or bandage is secure. If possible, try to get the casualty to support the injured arm or hand because it will help keep his or her mind off the injury.

Make sure bandages are not too tight

If possible, leave the casualty's fingertips or toes exposed when bandaging an arm or leg or applying a sling so that you can check that the blood circulation has not been affected by the bandage. Check the circulation in the affected area immediately after applying the bandage by pressing one of the nails in the bandaged limb until it turns white, then release the pressure. The nail should become pink again immediately. If colour does not return, or the fingers or toes look blue or feel unnaturally cold, the bandage is too tight. Remove the bandage immediately and reapply.

DRESSINGS

There are two main types of dressing: adhesive dressings and sterile dressings. *Adhesive dressings* are normally used to cover small injuries such as cuts and grazes; *sterile dressings* are used to protect large or serious wounds. Whichever dressing is used, the pad touching the wound MUST be larger than the wound.

ADHESIVE DRESSING

Also known as a "plaster", this type of dressing consists of a small absorbent pad of gauze or cellulose attached to an adhesive backing. Adhesive dressings come in a variety of shapes and sizes. Each one is sterilised and sealed in an individual packet.

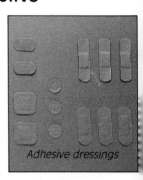
Adhesive dressings

WHAT TO DO

1 Wash the wound and dry the surrounding skin (see p. 79). Take the dressing out of its wrapping and hold it over the wound, gauze side down.

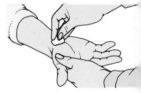

2 Peel back the protective strips but do not remove them. Without touching the pad with your fingers, carefully place the dressing over the wound.

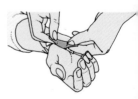

3 Gently pull the protective strips back completely and press the edges of the dressing down firmly.

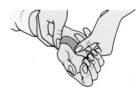

STERILE DRESSING

This dressing consists of layers of gauze and a pad of cotton wool attached to an open-weave gauze roller bandage. Each dressing is sterilised and wrapped in two protective wrappings. Avoid using this type of dressing if either seal is broken because it will not be sterile.

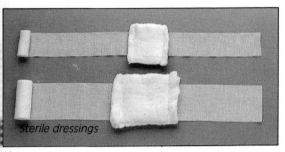

Sterile dressings

WHAT TO DO

1 Remove the outer wrappings and, without touching the gauze pad, hold the edge of the folded dressing and the rolled bandage in one hand and unfold the short end of the bandage with the other hand.

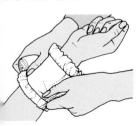

2 Place the pad gauze-side down on the wound. Do not touch the pad, although if the pad is folded, you can guide it by placing your fingers along its edge.

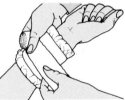

3 Wind the short end of the bandage once around the wound to secure the pad and leave it hanging free.

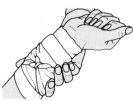

4 Bandage firmly using the rolled part of the bandage; tie both ends together over the pad using a **reef knot** (see p. 89).

85

ROLLER BANDAGES

Roller bandages are used to support a muscle or joint injury or to secure dressings and help maintain pressure to control bleeding. They are made in a variety of widths and lengths to fit different parts of the body. Crepe and conforming bandages are useful because they are stretchy and mould to the shape of the body.

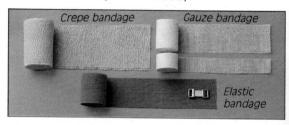

Crepe bandage   *Gauze bandage*

Elastic bandage

Rules for applying bandages
- Always stand in front of the casualty.
- Support the affected limb in the position in which it is to remain.
- Make sure the bandage is tightly rolled.
- Always work from below the injury up the limb and from the inner side of the limb outward.

WHAT TO DO

1 Hold the bandage with the rolled part uppermost, place the end of the bandage on the limb immediately below the injured area and make two straight turns.

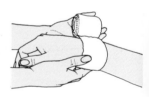

2 Working up the limb, make a series of spiral turns allowing each successive turn to cover two-thirds of the previous one.

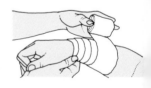

3 Finish off by making a straight turn around the limb, fold the end of the bandage over and secure it with a safety pin or bandage clip or as shown opposite.

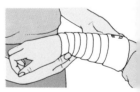

HAND/FOOT BANDAGE

WHAT TO DO

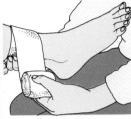

1 Make one straight turn around the casualty's ankle to secure the end of the bandage.

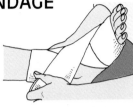

3 Make two straight turns around the ball of the casualty's foot. Carry the bandage back across the top of the foot to the ankle.

4 Continue making figure-of-eight turns around the foot and ankle. Make sure that each layer covers two-thirds of the previous one.

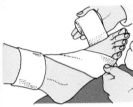

2 Take the bandage across the top of the foot to the base of the little toe, carry it under the ball of the foot and bring it up at the base of the casualty's big toe.

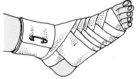

5 Finish off by making two straight turns around the ankle and secure the bandage.

Securing a roller bandage

Always fasten the end of a roller bandage with a safety pin or bandage clip if possible but if neither is available, secure it as shown.

Tying the bandage
Leave 15cm (6in) or more bandage free and cut it down the middle. Tie a knot at the bottom of the split. Wrap the ends around the limb and tie them.

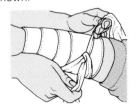

TRIANGULAR BANDAGES

Triangular bandages are normally made from un-bleached calico. They are used to support limbs with broken bones either folded as broad- or narrow-fold bandages (see below) or open as slings (see pp. 92–3), or to secure light dressings where pressure is not required (see pp. 90–1).

If you do not have a triangular bandage, you can make one by cutting a 1m (1yd) square piece of firmly woven fabric in half diagonally.

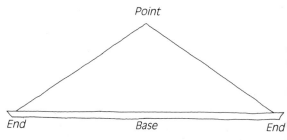

Point

End *Base* *End*

Open bandage
When using a triangular bandage as a sling, for example, keep the bandage open but fold up a narrow hem along the longest edge – the base.

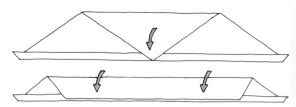

Broad-fold bandage
Used to secure broken legs (see p. 38) or for extra support after applying a sling (see p. 42). Fold a narrow hem along the base as above, fold the point to the base then fold the bandage in half again.

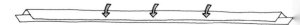

Narrow-fold bandage
This is used to tie the ankles and feet together when a casualty has an injured leg (see p. 38 and 40). Prepare a broad-fold bandage then fold the bandage in half again.

TYING A REEF KNOT

Always use a reef knot to secure the ends of a bandage because it will not slip, it will lie flat and will therefore be more comfortable for the casualty. A reef knot is also easy to undo.

When the knot is complete, tuck the ends in neatly and make sure that no part of the knot is pressing against the casualty. If necessary, place a pad or material or cotton wool under the knot.

WHAT TO DO

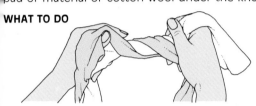

1 Take one end of the bandage in each hand. Take the right end of the bandage over the left end and pass it underneath.

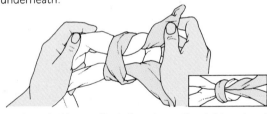

2 Bring what is now the left end over the right end and pass it under again. Pull the knot tight and tuck the ends in neatly.

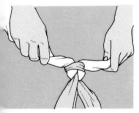

3 To untie a reef knot, take one pair of bandage ends as near to the knot as possible and pull them away from the knot.

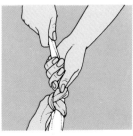

4 Slip the knot apart by sliding one of the ends through the knot.

TRIANGULAR BANDAGES *(continued)*

SCALP BANDAGE

WHAT TO DO

1 Fold a narrow hem along the *base* of a triangular bandage.

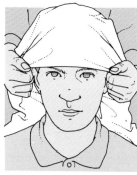

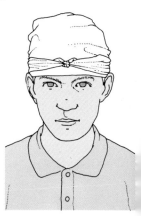

2 Place the centre of the *base* on the centre of the casualty's forehead just above his eyebrows and let the *point* hang down the back of his head and neck.

4 Tie the *ends* in a **reef knot** (see p. 89) on the centre of the casualty's forehead above his nose as close to the hem as possible.

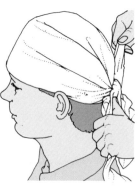

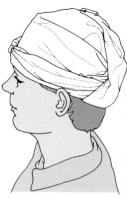

3 Carry the *ends* around the back of his head, cross them over the *point* then bring them around to the front.

5 Steady the casualty's head and gently pull the *point* down to take up the slack in the bandage. Carry the *point* up and pin it to the bandage on top of his head.

FOOT BANDAGE

WHAT TO DO

1 Lay a triangular bandage on the floor and fold a narrow hem along the *base*.

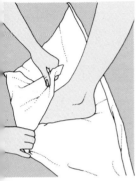

2 Place the casualty's foot on the bandage so that the base comes approximately half way up his ankle.

3 Bring the *point* of the bandage up over the casualty's toes – without bending them – and across the top of his foot.

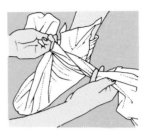

4 Pick up the *ends* of the bandage and carry them forward. Cross them over the front of the foot, take them around to the back of the ankle and cross them. Tie off in the front with a **reef knot** (see p. 89).

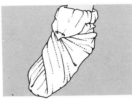

5 Take the *point* down over the top of the knot and secure it to the rest of the bandage with a safety pin.

Hand bandage

Use the same technique to secure a hand dressing but if the hand is very small, fold a deeper hem at the base of the bandage.

Applying the bandage
Place the hand, dressing side up, on the bandage so that the base of the bandage is level with the wrist and secure it as above.

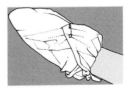

TRIANGULAR BANDAGES *(continued)*

ARM SLING

Arm slings are used to support an injured arm or to immobilise an upper limb in the case of a chest injury (see p. 40).

WHAT TO DO

1 Sit the casualty down, place her arm across her chest and ask her to support her arm; she may need help.

2 Using the space between the casualty's arm and elbow, ease a triangular bandage into place so that the *base* hangs down her body as shown, and the *point* extends beyond her elbow.

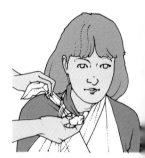

4 Bring the bottom *end* up over the arm to the neck and tie the ends in a **reef knot** (see p. 89) in the hollow above the casualty's collar bone.

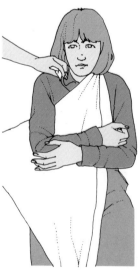

3 Take the top *end* of the bandage around the casualty's neck to the front again.

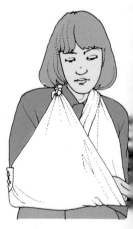

5 Tuck the excess bandage in behind the elbow, then bring the point forward and secure it to the front of the sling with a safety pin.

ELEVATION SLING

This sling is used to support an injured hand in a well-raised position to help control bleeding or to immobilise an arm if the collar bone is broken or several ribs are broken.

WHAT TO DO

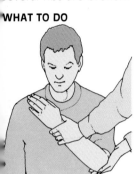

1 Place the arm on the injured side across the casualty's chest so that his fingertips almost touch the opposite shoulder.

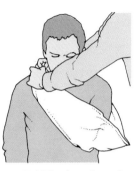

3 Fold the *base* in under the casualty's forearm and elbow and take the lower *end* around his back up over the other shoulder; tie off with a reef knot (see p. 89).

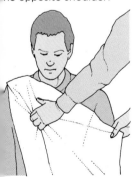

2 Place an open bandage over the casualty's arm so that the *base* of the bandage is down his body, one *end* is over his shoulder and the *point* reaches beyond his elbow.

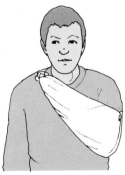

4 Tuck the *point* in between the forearm and the front of the bandage and turn the fold up over the casualty's arm and secure it to the sling with a safety pin.

IMPROVISED DRESSINGS AND BANDAGES

You should always use the correct dressings or bandages if they are available. However, if there is no first-aid kit, do not waste time looking for equipment: improvise as described below.

EMERGENCY DRESSINGS

If you have no dressings, use any clean non-fluffy material such as a handkerchief, pillow-case or paper tissue instead.

Wash your hands then hold the material by its corners and let it fall open. Re-fold it to the required size so that what was the inside, un-exposed surface is now the outside. Handle the dressing by the edges and place it over the wound immediately. Secure the dressing with a folded scarf; tie a **reef knot** over the pad (see p. 83).

IMPROVISED SLINGS

If there are no triangular bandages, there are several ways to support an injured arm while you take the casualty to hospital.

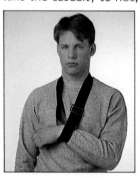

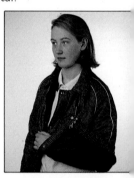

Using a belt or tie
You can support the arm with a belt, tie, braces or pair of tights tied around the casualty's neck. *Do not use this method if the forearm is injured.*

Folding up a jacket
For an injured forearm, turn the bottom of a jacket up over the injured arm and pin it to the top of the jacket.

INDEX

ACKNOWLEDGMENTS

Illustrators Jim Robins, Kevin Maddison

Photography Paul Fletcher, Karen Norquay

Typesetting Cambrian Typesetters